VEGAN
FREAK

being vegan in a non-vegan world

Bob Torres, PhD
Jenna Torres, PhD

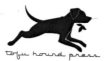

tofu hound press

First Printing 2005

Tofu Hound Press
PO Box 276
Colton, NY 13625-0276
publications@tofuhound.com

Sign up for updates from the publisher and explore our forthcoming titles at
http://tofuhound.com
Updates to the resources explored in this book are available at
http://veganfreak.com

ATTENTION VEGETARIAN CLUBS AND ORGANIZATIONS, CORPORATIONS, UNIVERSITIES, COLLEGES, AND PROFESSIONAL ORGANIZATIONS: Quantity discounts are available on bulk purchases of this book for educational, gift purposes, or as premiums for increasing magazine subscriptions or renewals. Special books or book excerpts can also be created to fit specific needs. Vegetarian clubs and organizations can also receive special volume discounts for this title, particularly if used for fund-raising purposes. For more information, please contact Tofu Hound Press, PO Box 276, Colton, NY 13625-0276; 315-262-0372; email: publications@tofuhound.com.

Text layout by Tofu Hound Press

Cover design and photography by Chad Miller / Fourteen Little Men, Inc.
www.fourteenlittlemen.com

ISBN 0-9770804-1-2

For Dan
the original commie vegan freak.

For Michi and Mole
the cat and dog who remind us everyday why we're vegan.

Acknowledgments

Thanks to **Dan Peyser** of thesmokingvegan.blogspot.com in the Burlington office of Tofu Hound Press. This book would truly not be what it is without his editing, advice, ideas, and suggestions. We'd probably also not be vegans were it not for his patient help. We can't thank you enough, Dan.

Thanks to our brilliant reviewers, **Gary Loewenthal** of animalwritings.com, **Theresa Petray**, **Chris and Ginger Sweeney**, and **Lindsay Timmerman**. All of your advice, ideas, and suggestions certainly made the work stronger. And Lindsay, you're a completely fucking wicked copy editor. You rock.

Our dog and cat had a central role in the production of this book. **Michi** (the cat) specialized in blocking monitors, kitty-typing, and sitting on manuscripts being edited. **Mole**, our dog, mostly tried to eat rough drafts and had some kind of weird attachment to sniffing the cables on the back of Bob's PowerMac G4. We also came up with most of the rough ideas for the book while walking the dog in the woods near our house.

We're also grateful for **students** who have given us much to think about. The local **Vegan Action Group** and students in Bob's **class on animal rights** in Spring 2005 were especially helpful.

Of course, we gotta thank **our parents** for putting up with us, for tirelessly promoting the book, and for being cool about our veganism. *Can you please not read the section on sex toys? Thanks.*

Chad Miller of Fourteen Little Men designed our excellent cover. He captured exactly what we were after even though we were probably vague as hell. He's amazingly talented, and we appreciate his hard work.

Thanks to **Isa Chandra Moskowitz** of the Post Punk Kitchen for writing the foreword for us and being enthusiastic about this project. Her cookbook *Vegan With a Vengeance* should be out Fall 2005. Go buy a thousand copies. The recipes are completely brilliant. We need more vegans like Isa!

Finally, thanks to **all of our readers** over at VeganFreaks.org for the comments and ideas on things we've posted there. Many of you have helped us to see things in a new light.

Table of Contents

Foreword

Is it any coincidence that Vegans are not only a group of people who prefer not to consume any animal products but also a science fiction species from a planet inhabiting the star system Vega?

I don't think so.

Sometimes it feels like we are indeed aliens and this "Planet Earth" we've landed on is not a welcoming one. The creatures are not waving white flags and approaching us with a gentle curiosity, bearing gifts of fruit from their world and marveling at how we can be so different yet the same. Rather, the townsfolk come out guns blazing and torches ignited, shouting "Plants have feelings!" and preparing for their own brand of vigilante justice. Only we aren't aliens. Mostly we are just common townsfolk like them and try as we might to explain ourselves they won't put down the torches long enough to listen.

Sometimes being vegan is like that. And that's where *Vegan Freak* steps in. Part etiquette (how do we deal with Uncle Jake's meat jokes?), part strategy (what is the most effective argument when he tells us that plants have feelings) and part survival (aisles and aisles of food and nothing to eat?!), *Vegan Freak: being vegan in a non-vegan world* is a handbook for the terrain on this strange new planet.

The desire to not cause undue harm to animals (including humans) is a natural one, and most people have felt sparks of this at some point in their lives. Vegans have just taken this feeling to its logical conclusion. *Vegan Freak* makes that connection and in turn helps us to be able to make the connection with other people. I admit when I first received the manuscript I thought "But I already know everything there is to know about veganism!" Well that may be so—or maybe I'm just belligerent— but *Vegan Freak* is a must read for vegans, most of all because it is written for us, the people who are already there. *Vegan Freak* helps to keep us there, and helps us to deal with the hurdles of the rest of the world not being there with us. It is a must read for vegetarians who are on the fence and haven't taken the leap. And it is just as valuable for those curious about veganism since most questions I have ever been asked are answered here.

foreword

The thing that struck me most about *Vegan Freak* is that it made me realize being vegan is actually easy. We have plenty of food to choose from, plenty of cruelty-free companies to purchase from and plenty of people to support us along the way.

When I finished reading, I was prepared to get in my spaceship and fly back home, but then I realized I already was home.

Anyone interested in buying a used spaceship?

Isa Chandra Moskowitz

author of *Vegan with a Vengeance : 125 Delicious, Cheap, Animal-Free, Logo-Free Recipes That Rock*

New York, NY

July 2005

"Auschwitz begins wherever someone looks at a slaughterhouse and thinks: they're only animals."
-Theodor Adorno

The world only goes forward because of those who oppose it.
– Goethe

chapter one:
vegan
and freaky

"A vegan is someone who, for various reasons, chooses to avoid using or consuming animal products. While vegetarians choose not to use flesh foods, vegans also avoid dairy and eggs, as well as fur, leather, wool, down, and cosmetics or chemical products tested on animals." –Vegan Action (http://www.vegan.org)

All vegans have been there—if you're vegan, you know the situation well. Perhaps it's at work. Maybe it's with friends or even family. You sit down to eat, quietly ordering a salad or the ubiquitous (and so very tired) grilled vegetable entree, and some observant dinner companion notices that you're not chowing down on the chicken smothered in cream sauce and butter topped with bacon, or whatever the heart attack Atkins®–approved special du jour is. You are keeping to yourself, completely quiet and proper, and suddenly, in that moment of omnivorous realization, without any work on your part, you're turned into the militant animal rights activist, earthy weirdo, and transcender of all that is good and righteous in the world.

In short, you've become The Vegan Freak.

vegan freak

All of us who are vegan have at some time or another just felt like absolute outsiders in the places that we're supposed to be the most comfortable: our homes, our jobs, and with our friends and families. Though most vegans are likely not any "freakier" than your average person, we like to use the term "freak" here because the simple and compassionate act of denying animal products for ethical reasons can make you into the weirdo at the dinner table or in other social and personal contexts. You're the alien visiting from Vega, great rejector of convention and all that is good and right in the world. Even if you're not a preachy and self-righteous 'vegangelical,' you can still get the looks and their accompanying huffs of displeasure and eye-rolls; you're still the object of anything from curiosity to outright hostility, and people still look at you like you you've sprouted a third eye on your forehead when you mention veganism.

Though you may wonder how we expect to sell a book that seems to insult our very audience by calling them freaks, we're hoping you can proudly claim, embrace, and use your vegan freakdom. This is the first step towards vegan freak pride, and it's a step towards keeping you a happy vegan and building solid vegan community. We've also written this book because we know how it is to be vegan and to be thought of as freaky. We want to help you through it, or at least help you to embrace it, particularly if you're a new vegan or just contemplating veganism. As contrarians at heart, we have little problem with being regarded this way, even if it does become tiresome on occasion. Still, we consider ourselves pretty lucky—we have a good support network of vegan friends to lean on and commiserate with. Yet as we know from our blog at veganfreaks.org, there are many of you out there who don't have such a solid support network or friends to help you through what has been called "the vegan blues."

One of our main goals in writing this book is to help ease the transition for new vegans or those contemplating veganism. When we became vegan, we noticed there were precious few sources that dealt with the everyday ins-and-outs of veganism. Not all of us are fortunate enough to live in a community with other vegans, and for those of you that don't know another vegan, how do you ever find out about the practical everyday stuff of veganism? A lot of us muddle through it, not really sure how to deal with anything beyond not eating or using animal products, and we learn as we go. Sometimes, we learn as we go with painful consequences (like, say, learning the hard way that Thanksgiving dinner probably isn't the time to talk about factory farming and animal oppression). Perhaps you're in a different spot: maybe you're thinking about becoming a vegan but you think it is too hard, too impractical, or a social mess. You would be a vegan right now if you could just figure out how to tell your parents, or if you could put up with your jeering friends, or maybe you're thinking about it and just want to know more. The advice, ideas, and experience that you'll find in this book should help.

At this point, we know how some of you vegans out there are responding. You're likely pissed at us already because we're making veganism sound "hard." Let's be clear: we think becoming a vegan is actually pretty easy. In terms of major changes in your life and your perception of the world, it is likely one of the easier things that you'll do. On top of that, the rewards are ample, which we'll get into below. But because of the way food and our food choices are so intimately linked to who we are and how we're perceived, sometimes being a vegan can be a pain —not because of you living by your choices, but because of the way people react to them. It can also sometimes be hard to be a vegan in a world set up to cater to choices you have real moral, ethical, or political gripes with. Think about it: when was the last time you saw a drive-thru or fast food restaurant that served whole-grain vegan foods?

If you're not used to it, it can also be difficult to suddenly be thought of as a "radical" as you shift towards veganism. In his excellent (and highly recommended!) book *Empty Cages,* Tom Regan talks about the ways in which folks concerned about animal rights are painted as violent, terrorist radicals by the media and by the animal cruelty industries. Against this stereotype perpetuated by the media, Regan writes that most people concerned with animal rights are actually "Norman Rockwell Americans." Though we're not sure that pierced, tattooed Latino vegans like Bob count as "Norman Rockwell Americans," we do get what he means, and we think it is powerful. What he's saying is that a growing interest on your part in animal rights doesn't suddenly mean that tomorrow you're going to join the Animal Liberation Front, hurl Molotov cocktails at research facilities, and threaten researchers. Regan says that most people who come to consciousness about animal rights are "just ordinary folks." As you shift into veganism for ethical reasons, people might suddenly think of you as different, though you may not have changed all that much. Like it or not, you have to deal with this, regardless of how you feel about radical actions on behalf of animal liberation. Some non-vegans are open-minded, cool beyond belief, and ready to accept you for who you are. Others will view you with deep suspicion, tagging you a freak (at best) or an anti-American radical (at worst). In the pages that follow, we'll give you some advice about how to deal with this.

One of our main ideas in writing this book is that we think the transition to veganism should be as easy as possible. Though both radical and non-radical tactics are important for fighting animal exploitation, veganism is the first necessary step one should take towards ending animal oppression. By being vegan, you send an important message, both symbolically and practically. Symbolically, you remind people why eating meat is problematic, and that's important. Carol Adams says that when you practice veganism, you're essentially "standing in" for the animal who's now a thing (food) and no longer present. Your very presence and choices remind people—however subtly—that the death of animals for pure enjoyment is wrong (and since it is possible to live very well as a vegan, eating animals is nothing more than death for the sake of taste). Practically, you're withdrawing your support of an industry that kills at least 8 billion animals a year in the United States alone. Though there are few vegans, our impact can be great. If you become a vegan around age 20 or so, your choice will keep something like 2000-3000 animals out of the slaughterhouse. Thinking about it this way, if we can help just a few of you to become vegan or stay vegan, then together, we'll have done something remarkably effective towards helping to end the outright misery factory farm animals endure.

Another plus is that veganism can be contagious. When thoughtful people around you come to understand you as a sensible person who's making committed and ethical choices, they begin to think about their own choices, and some of them become vegans or vegetarians as a result. Just living your everyday life as a vegan, you can be a powerful multiplier! Not to mention, as an additional vegan-plus, there's more and more evidence a diet rich in whole-grain plant foods is good for you[1]. By being a vegan, you can not only improve your health, you can also help to end needless animal exploitation.

And, on top of that, being vegan just plain rocks. If you drive by cows at pasture, you can now look at them knowing that you aren't responsible for their exploitation and death. We've spoken to lots of vegans, and many have agreed that our relationship with animals changes as a result of our ethical choices. Finally, the kind of consciousness you bring to being vegan can also seep into other parts of your life.

The Health Nut and the Hippie

We know there are guides out there that tell you how to be a healthy, happy vegan, but we think our book is of a different sort, and likely appeals to a different audience. We're dork academic professor types (at least that's what we do to pay the bills), and so when we want to understand something, we devour books on the topic. When we got into veganism, we read just about everything we could get our hands on (and we're still reading). After doing all of this reading, we found out that many of the books on the day-to-day details of veganism tend to fall into two camps: the health nut and the hippie (or both). Now, before you health nuts and hippies get mad at us, let us make some

---

1. See T. Colin Campbell's latest book *The China Study* for one of the latest studies on this topic.

disclaimers. First, we should say that we don't have any problem with people who are concerned about their health. We're concerned about our health too. We try to eat well, and the health-based arguments for veganism are scientifically solid and well beyond proven. Second, we should say that we love all you hippies too...every stinkin', drum-beating, dead-head one of you. Just kidding. We really do like hippies. Some of our best friends are hippies.

For us, as we were getting into veganism, we wanted more than the health-based arguments, or pages upon pages about vitamin B12, or even how to eat if you're a vegan athlete. These are important things, no doubt, but there are already quite a few books that do these things particularly well (see Appendix B or our website for suggested reading). Also, we wanted more than the spiritual, earth-mother stuff. Yes, respecting the lives of animals is good spiritual practice, likely good for your karma, and completely solid for the health of the earth, but sometimes books in this vein strike us as a bit too new-agey for our tastes. It was like the audience for these books was a bit more into chakra alignment than we were. We wanted a book that spoke to people like us: young, with punk-ish/radical leanings, and primarily into veganism for ethics and animal rights. We wanted an author that wasn't afraid to be irreverent or to say "fuck," or to tease hippies in good fun. When we realized that there wasn't a book like what we wanted, we decided that we had to write our own, and here we are.

In this book, we've collected all of those little tips that we found incredibly useful when we became vegans. It took us a pretty long time to come up with some of these things, and we learned some hard lessons along the way. We want you to benefit from our experience and our mistakes.

Going Vegan: The Cold Tofu Approach

If you are an ovo-lacto vegetarian who isn't yet a vegan and you're looking for advice for going vegan, our advice is simple: stop eating animal products today, and give it three weeks before you decide that you *must* go back to eating dairy and eggs. If your commitment to animals is strong, is three weeks without cheese that much to give for the cause? Three weeks isn't much when you think about it. It is just 21 quick days. That's 7 days fewer than it took zombies to take over the UK in *28 Days Later* (or, if you prefer cheesy movies, that's 7 fewer days than it took the character that no-talent Sandra Bullock played to get clean in *28 Days*). 21 days is less time than you'd have to spend as a contestant on the average crappy reality TV show. Do you have a tattoo? If you do, it took your tattoo longer than 21 days to heal.

Point is, 21 days isn't much, but it is enough time for you to prove to yourself that life is easy to live without animal products–and trust us, it is. Going "cold tofu" (har!) is actually easier than weaning yourself off of animal products by gradually reducing the amount you eat over time. To take an example, let's say you *really* love cheese. In your mind, you imagine that life without your beloved cheese would be like life without sunny days, cute puppies, and chocolate (or in Bob's case, sunny days, cute puppies, and cold beer). If you decide to phase it out by eating only a little each day, you're actually giving the thing you're working to consume less and less of *even more power.* If you plan on phasing out cheese over 3 or 4 months, you'll eventually look forward to even the tiniest bit of it, as if it were some reward. On the other hand, if you go "cold tofu," you may tremble and suffer like an addict in withdrawal for a day or two, but after that, the suffering will decrease. By day 20, cheese might even look nasty to you. Or, perhaps, you'll be a lifelong non-cheesing cheeseaholic. (Yeah, that was cheesy).

Don't be all vegan-hatin' on us. Just try it for three weeks. What do you have to lose except products that make animals suffer?

How We Went Vegan

We used the above three week method to go vegan and kick our animal product habits, but sadly, it took us a while to get to a point where we even considered veganism possible. Looking back, once we made the decision to do it, going vegan was easy for us, but getting there was another story.

It took us a long time to see veganism as possible and desirable. Longer than it should have. Like, much longer than it should have. As in years. When we weren't vegans, it seemed to us that vegans we knew emerged from their mothers' wombs pre-veganized or something, complete with a vegan gene, a V chromosome, or some other modern day mystery of biochemistry that suppressed their desire for meat, eggs, dairy, wool, and leather. Though some vegans are vegans from the day they come into the world, the vast majority of us aren't born vegan, and when you're a cheese- and egg-eating vegetarian or a meat-eater, veganism looks tough from afar—tougher than it is.

Part of what we do for fun is ask vegans we know how they became vegan. The stories of how people come to their vegan consciousness are almost always intriguing. For some people, it is like a brilliant flash of inspiration. For others, it takes a long time of kicking things around and basically just trying to figure out where they're heading and what they're doing. Here, we share our pathways to veganism. Maybe you'll find something familiar in them, maybe not.

Bob on How He Became Vegan

One of the things that amazes me about myself is my ability to suppress information I don't want to think about for some reason or another. I think the touchy-feely self-help types and my friends who've been to therapy call this "denial." I can deny with the best of them, and I can think myself into or out of just about anything with enough effort. Global warming? Feh, I can't do much about it. Republican domination of national politics? Feh, they're only a little worse than the Dems. The fact that I'm writing a book that will never get me tenure? Feh, there's more to life than work. Animals being used for meat, leather, wool, and experimentation? Feh, the world will never change.

Or at least that's what I used to think until something hit me, and it hit me hard. I couldn't just suppress it, deny it, or pretend that it'd go away. I'd woken up to a unique form of consciousness that many vegans get to if they're going to stay vegan. I stepped away from seeing animals as ours to use and instead starting seeing them as beings who deserved respect. There were a number of things that did this for me, but a little trip into my biography might be helpful here.

As a child, particularly up until I was about 10, I was something of a loner. I spent a lot of time with my dog, but didn't have many human friends my age. Spending all this time with my pound mutt Patches was fundamental for me in how I evolved my feelings about animals. I loved my dog dearly. She was my closest friend for a very long time, and we were virtually inseparable. Around this time, in my youthful fantasies, I also entertained thoughts of being a veterinarian, and I used to pretend I was the "wilderness doctor" who would save sick animals. From pretty early on, I felt a connection to animals, but it took what seems like an eternity for me to realize that the connection had to go deeper than just loving pets.

When I started high school, I attended a magnet vo-tech school in the Philadelphia public school system that devoted a few periods of each day to animal care, plant science, and horticulture. During high school, I had the chance to work more closely with animals and plants, and I began to learn even more about rearing animals and agriculture in general. After high school, I went to Penn State University, where I double-majored in Philosophy and Agricultural Science. Philosophy gave me the intellectual stimulation of figuring out difficult theoretical puzzles and making solid arguments, while Agricultural Science provided me with more training in animal husbandry, plant science, and other aspects of modern agricultural production I became interested in during my vo-tech days. It was as an ag-sci major that I learned about "modern" techniques of factory farming and how despicable they really were. In the courses I took, I learned that animals were "economic units" who had a certain "useful" lifespan. Once this economically productive lifespan was over, the animals became less profitable and had to be slaughtered. Taking classes on agricultural production, I saw how animals on contemporary factory farms were treated, how they suffered, and how they were often mutilated—without anesthetics—as routine parts of a long process designed to produce the cheapest possible meat, eggs, and dairy. The sad part is that this kind of production was considered to be state-of-the-art, while less torturous forms of production were considered to be old-fashioned, economically unscalable, and non-competitive. The more I learned, the more I knew that animal agriculture was wrong. I realized that our cheap meat was coming at the price of tremendous suffering, and I couldn't be a party to that.

It was around this time, probably during my third year in college or so, that a copy of John Robbins' *Diet for a New America* fell into my lap. I devoured the book and decided that the only real option for me was to become a vegetarian. From that point on, I was a pretty solid ovo-lacto vegetarian for 6 or 7 years. Somehow, over that time, I think my vegetarianism became less of a conscious decision for me and more of a habit. In time, I began to forget why I was a vegetarian. As a result, I did something that now makes me nearly insane: I'd very occasionally eat meat, usually on holidays or on vacation. As I look back, part of this had to do with wanting to please others and not be a pain, part of it was sheer laziness, and part of it was that I'd stopped being completely aware of why I was a vegetarian. (See, there's that denial working its way back into the picture.) I also publicly supported vegans, but quietly thought they went too far. At the time, painting vegans as out-there weirdos (and that's saying something coming from an out-there weirdo like me) was one of the denial tactics I used to keep myself guilt-free about my decisions. I figured vegans were marginal radicals, and in so figuring, I was able to minimize their actions in my mind. This absurd preconception was also aided by a few run-ins over the years with proselytizing, nasty vegans who seemed hell-bent on lecturing, chiding, and berating me for being a vegetarian.

Once I started teaching, however, I did a section in one of my classes on meat, vegetarianism, and ethics. I reminded myself why I was a vegetarian, and grew to appreciate the vegan perspective. As a New Year's resolution, I renewed my commitment to ovo-lacto vegetarianism, and stuck with it. Newly invigorated as a vegetarian, I decided to further explore the question of animal rights, and I started reading tons of books on ethical theory. I read *Animal Liberation* by Peter Singer and I was struck by the logic of his argument for veganism. Here was someone who appealed not to cute little animals, but to reason. His points were solid. His logic was (largely) impeccable[2] and I decided then and there that animal exploitation was just plain wrong in any form. There was no reason—beyond my own simple pleasure at the taste of milk, cheese, and eggs—that animals should die for me, or for any of us. If I was going to be true to myself and live by my ethics, what choice did I have but to go the extra step and give up dairy and eggs? As someone who cared about animal rights, I was nothing more than a hypocrite if I continued to consume dairy and eggs, particularly because of the amount of death and suffering involved. For those unconvinced: when dairy cows become less "productive," they're sent to slaughter. Period. There's no nice little pasture somewhere that retired cows end up on, unless you consider ground beef a 'nice pasture.' Those who eat dairy products are directly supporting the meat industry and not limiting suffering terribly much (this goes for organic milk too). Similarly, the production of eggs is incomprehensibly cruel. Multiple egg laying chickens are stacked in a small wire box for their entire lives, they see little daylight, and they rarely, if ever, get to even flap their wings or move freely (we discuss all of this in the next chapter).

So, I did what I had to do: I stopped eating animal products of any kind, and began to phase out all other animal products or animal-tested products from my life, including things like shampoos, lotions, and even—dread—condoms (more on this later). In a few years, I went from thinking that vegans were excessive, marginal weirdos who had nothing better to do than lecture well-meaning vegetarians to being a vegan myself. I'm glad that I was able to see past my initial misconceptions.

---

2. Though I'm still a big fan of Peter Singer and I appreciate what he's done for the cause of animal liberation, I've since discovered that his logic isn't necessarily the best out there. See Appendix B for more suggestions on reading in this area.

An oft-repeated cliché (so oft-repeated I hesitate to use it) is that no man is an island, and that's true enough in this case. Three things came together at the same time for me that helped me see that veganism was the only choice for me. First, I was fortunate enough to have Jenna to talk to about my evolving change in consciousness, and together, we decided to go vegan, which helped a great deal. Second, we were fortunate enough to be "like, totally BFF"[3] with Dan Peyser (to whom this book is partly dedicated), a vegan, communist student of mine from Vermont who not only knew Marx better than anyone I've met before or since, but who also was completely patient, approachable, and cool with our questions about veganism. He made us feel comfortable talking to him about veganism, he never lectured or proselytized, and he gracefully put up with questions that personally now drive me mad in my less patient moments. For example, before I came to the realization that I had to become vegan to be true to my principles, I'd tell Dan that I'd be vegan "except for cream in my coffee." I think I also wondered aloud to him how I'd ever eat pizza without cheese, what I'd do without yogurt, and how I'd miss diner breakfasts if I became a vegan. Looking back at myself, I'm ashamed that I ever said these absurd things to Dan, and I realize how annoying I was, always coming at him with creative (yet poor) excuses about why I couldn't be vegan. I did the very things to Dan that I complain about almost daily. *Dan, if you're reading, I owe you man—big time. How did you not throttle me?*

Much of this also coincides with us getting a new puppy, which is the third driver in this whole vegan move in our lives. Though we had a cat for many years, the cat is a relatively independent creature. Sure, he needs his daily dose of love, but more often than not, I have the sense that I'm invading his privacy, his beauty sleep, and/or his territory. He's a lover and a lovely, chunky, happy cat, who we love dearly but he's a cat – and it is in his nature to be, well, cat-like. Getting a puppy, however, is a different kind of experience. Puppies are needy in ways that kittens

---

3. For those of you not in the know, this is how I'm told that teenage girls communicate who their best friends are (BFF = Best Friends Forever)

are not. When we brought the dog home, he was only a few weeks old and completely dependent on us. I spent about three weeks solid with the puppy, taking the place of his mother, and raising him as though he were my own 4–legged furry child. In doing this, we developed a real bond with him. Like the cat, we came to see him as a member of our family, and knew his moods, his wants, and what made him happy. Similarly, I think he learned to see these things in us as well, and we grew together. Knowing both the cat and the dog had such a wide range of emotions from fear to sadness to complete and total joy, we figured other animals must also experience similar feelings. From my studies, I knew that pigs were at least as smart as dogs, that cows recognized people they saw frequently, and that chickens were more than "stupid birds." Why, we wondered, should our dog and cat be treated like royalty while other animals suffered horrible fates? Though we couldn't stop animal agriculture immediately, we did realize that being vegan was a way for us to remove our support for this exploitative, cruel, and unfair hierarchy of animal oppression. After that, my awareness of animal rights grew even beyond the "cute fluffies" of dogs and cats.

Since becoming vegan, I haven't looked back, and I've had no regrets whatsoever. Milk, cheese, and eggs now seem kind of nasty to me, and I have no desire to eat them at all. I view animals differently, seeing more of a kinship than anything else. I also see my place in society somewhat differently. Though I'm not a hectoring "vegangelical" like those who have turned me off in the past, I like to think my choices serve as a simple reminder that there's something morally objectionable to eating meat. I can do this even without saying a single word about veganism, because, like we said at the start of this chapter, people notice what you eat, and they wonder why you don't eat certain things. Our simple act of abstaining from animal products by choice reminds others that there are ethical problems in consuming animal products. This part of veganism is important to me, because even though it can create arguments, it also helps thoughtful people ask questions, think about why we'd be vegan, and possibly overcome their own denial about where our meat, dairy, and eggs come from and how much suffering is in every bite.

After all, if it worked for this world-class denier, it could probably work for anyone.

Jenna on How She Became Vegan

As I look back on my road to veganism, it strikes me that for most of my life I've been naive when it comes to how animals are treated, either because I didn't know the truth, or because I ignored the truth. As a kid, I was always kind of grossed out by meat. I would constantly pick at my food because I wanted to keep every last bit of mystery matter out of my mouth. (This took a lot of time and effort during meals, and annoyed my parents to no end.) Even though it grossed me out to see the veins in a chicken breast or the odd bits of fat and gristle on a pork chop, I ate the meat anyway. It tasted good, and after all, people are supposed to eat meat. It didn't even occur to me that there was an alternative.

As a kid, I was very interested in nature, but otherwise I'm not sure where I got my love for animals. Maybe it was all those *Ranger Rick* magazines or wildlife cards I got in the mail. Maybe it was that I always liked visiting the cows at my great-grandmother's farm. I did have some bad petting zoo experiences though, getting knocked over by a hungry goat who wanted to eat the entire cone full of food I had in my hand. I also never had any pets growing up, since my sister was severely allergic to cats and dogs, and my mom didn't like animals in the house. Because I could never have any pets, I eventually became fascinated with having one. It also helped that our family was adopted by our neighbor's cat, and I would surreptitiously let him in our house all the time so I could hang out with him. Knowing this cat well, however, did not stop me from dissecting a cat in 11th grade biology. At the time, I had no problems with the dissection because it was in the name of "science" (though I'm not sure what's so "scientific" about letting 11th graders tear apart cats for anatomy lessons). Today, I couldn't even fathom being in the same room with dissected animals.

Eventually, my love of nature and biology led me to major in plant science in college. As with so many people, I became much more aware of the world at this time in my life, and started getting interested in politics, concerned about the environmental impacts of our way of life, and appreciative of people different than me. I even met some vegetarians, and at the time, I didn't think they'd mind the chicken stock that I used to make the brown rice casserole that I brought to their potluck. (See, I was naive!) And as also happens to many people, I was unhealthy and overweight during college. I stopped exercising like I did in high school, I ate anything and everything, and drank a lot of (okay, too much) beer. As I got to my junior year I realized something needed to change. Luckily, Bob had a suggestion—we should become vegetarians. I thought he was crazy at first, since I never thought I could do it. I complained that it would be way too hard, although something in it appealed to me. Then he gave me *Diet for a New America* to read. That solidified it for me. We both went vegetarian (ovo-lacto), started cycling, lost 10 pounds, and became increasingly happy with this way of life.

Over the years, though, we became lazy vegetarians. We lost sight of why we became vegetarians in the first place, and started "cheating." After all, the occasional hot turkey sandwich smothered in gravy wouldn't hurt, right? We also got tired of trying to figure out what to do on holidays with family, and of eating salad or pasta primavera smothered in cream sauce in restaurants, and would just eat fish or chicken instead. A year living in Spain during graduate school definitely signified the end of our vegetarian ways. Even though we almost always cooked vegetarian at home, we thought we needed to eat meat to get the full cultural experience while eating out. When we got back, we tried to be mostly vegetarian but would still occasionally eat meat, mostly for the sake of saving face with friends (what a mistake that was!).

I have to admit that for the longest time I thought all vegans were freaks. As an ovo-lacto vegetarian, I didn't understand why the extra (and what I thought to be more difficult step) was necessary. No animals were killed for milk or eggs, right? Ah, how naive I was! Deep down, I did have a sense that something was not right with eating dairy and eggs, but I suppressed that feeling and kept merrily eating them.

Luckily, things change. Bob and I were at a point in our life again where we weren't happy with our diet. We were tired of cheating. We were tired of being semi-vegetarians. And we had another change in our life—we got a puppy. Even though we've had a cat since we started graduate school, having both animals at the same time made me realize how varied their emotions and personalities are. They are very different animals but they both learn, love, and show distinct emotions towards us. The dog and the cat helped me *finally* to make the connection to other animals—if I wouldn't eat or be cruel to my pets, I should never eat or be cruel to any other animal either. I didn't want to see any animals suffer on my behalf.

So, when Bob suggested we become vegans, this time I was completely ready and thinking about it myself before he even mentioned it. I read *Animal Liberation* by Peter Singer and *Mad Cowboy* by Howard Lyman, and just about everything else I could get my hands on related to animal rights, veganism, and health. I also need to give credit to our friend Dan Peyser, a "real live vegan" who opened our eyes to veganism. Getting to know Dan, I realized I had never really known any vegans that well before, and it was one of the reasons I had such a hard time considering the possibility. Dan never pushed the issue, but just showed us through his actions (and gentle reminders) that veganism is important and possible.

This time, I've gotten rid of any naive notions about animals. I've learned the truth about eggs and dairy, and I've taken it to heart. I initially had a few "but I'll miss cheese" moments, but I don't miss cheese at all! I am one happy vegan. I feel great physically, and I feel even better mentally knowing that I am not participating in the horrors of factory farming. I also like being part of a community dedicated to reducing suffering and cruelty to animals, humans, and the earth alike. Becoming vegan was one of the best decisions of my life, and I want to share that happiness with others through example and support.

Pathways to Veganism

Even though our stories are pretty similar, we know there are as many veganism "conversion" stories as there are vegans. People end up vegan for all kinds of reasons, and we love to hear how. If you feel like sharing yours with others, we encourage you to visit the forums on the companion website to this book at http://veganfreak.com and share how you came to veganism. Alternately, if you're not quite there yet, stop by and get some support for making the step (and in all honesty, it isn't as big a step as you'd think—trust us here!).

From our perspective, pretty much any pathway to veganism is a valid one. The more vegans, the better! Nevertheless, some people do go vegan for the wrong reasons, and as a result, many eventually become a special breed of annoyance, the "ex-vegan." If you've been a vegetarian or vegan for any time at all, you've surely met the disgruntled ex-vegetarian/vegan, the person who simply can't or won't give up bacon, fish, or whatever animal product they're deeply devoted to for the simple sake of taste. We'll talk more about ex-vegans and how to deal with them in Chapter 3. But for now, suffice it to say that ex-vegans are usually the by-product of poor reasons for turning vegan. As we see it, there are a bunch of wrong reasons to become vegan, but all of them revolve around one's heart, ethics, and principles not being at the core of this choice[4].

Fame and Friends

If someone has become a vegan because they're the biggest Moby fan on the planet and they, like, totally, must do like whatever Moby does, chances are that they're not becoming vegan for the right reasons. We admire Moby and what he does for the greater cause of veganism, but if someone is drawn to the cause simply because a celebrity supports it—and for no other reason—they're setting themselves up for a world

---

4. Thanks to Dan Peyser for neatly tying up some of these categories in his writing at *The Smoking Vegan* (http://thesmokingvegan.blogspot.com/). Some of what we've written in this section is based on his angry rants there.

of hurt. If your own heart isn't in the decision, odds are good it won't last long, and the last thing the world needs is another ex-vegan.

Similarly, if someone becomes vegan because all of their friends are doing it, they're likely not long-term vegans if they don't expand their consciousness beyond this basic reason.

Moral Superiority

Some people like being vegan so they can feel morally superior to meat-eaters and just about everyone else. These people strike a double-blow to veganism as a movement and cause: not only do they turn off potential vegans who aren't interested in being vegan police, they also send the message that all vegans are food Nazis hellbent on lecturing people on their food choices. Not eating meat *is* morally and ethically superior to supporting factory farming, but there's a time and place for this kind of discussion, and the quickest way to lose an audience is to call people murderers and stare down your nose at them.

Also, recall from our vegan "conversion" stories how important it was to us to know a vegan that was patient, supportive, and thoughtful. Wouldn't you rather be this kind of vegan?

Attention and Image (or, Slap Your Ass Instead)

Others become vegan because they think it is cool, different, and radical, and that it'll make them stand out and draw attention to them. For the record, there are easier and more effective ways to draw attention to yourself than going vegan. An old roommate of ours used to take great pleasure in pulling down his pants in front of people, bending over, and rhythm slapping his butt cheeks until they were a shiny, pimply red. This used to get him lots of attention, and we suspect that for some people, this is easier than veganism (though you might check with your local ordinances to see if this is legal where you live). The point of this ass-slapping diversion is to simply say that going vegan for image and attention is like getting a tattoo that you don't like. Sure, it can draw attention to you, but you're stuck living with it when everything is said and done.

But....

Yeah, there's always a but.

Some people can begin being vegans for the wrong reasons but then, by some stroke of luck, they can gain more awareness and become more solid in their veganism. We'd not deny there's some power in that kind of move. Generally, though, one's choice to go vegan needs to be more thoughtful than a simple bandwagon jump or attention grab. Veganism is undoubtedly the way forward on a number of fronts, but people must come to their own choices if they're to be meaningful for them. All we're saying is that when it comes down to it, the choice to be vegan must truly be yours or else it isn't likely something you'll stick with.

For those of you out there who might not yet be sure this is a choice you're ready to make, keep reading. In Chapter 2, we provide a basic primer on animal rights, factory farming, and the advantages of veganism for your health and the environment. If you're one of our non-vegan readers and not terribly convinced just yet, the debates and ideas in Chapter 2 will surely give you something to think about. Also, our appendices contains suggestions for further reading, and our website contains freshly updated links to blogs, forums, and other sites that can help both on-the-fence folks and vegans alike.

Regardless of whether you're vegan or just thinking about becoming vegan, it is important to remember that veganism isn't about complete perfection. No, we don't mean you should "cheat" and eat eggs and dairy. Read on, and you'll see what we mean.

Perfection and the Vegan Police

Veganism isn't about some saintly form of perfection—instead, being a vegan for ethical reasons is about reducing suffering to the greatest extent possible and practical, and it is up to you to define just how far that goes. We have our ideas about it (which you'll be reading soon), but ultimately, like the choice to be a vegan, you must live with your choices, so it is up to you to make them.

Newer vegans might be wondering what the trick is to veganism. Isn't ethical veganism[5] just about refusing animal products like meat, eggs, milk, and leather? Yes, this is surely the bedrock of ethical veganism, but if you go a bit further, it is possible to drive yourself completely insane thinking about the animal products present in the millions of things you'd never expect them to be in. Film contains gelatin. The tires in your car likely contain by-products of the animal slaughter industry. Your car itself probably has leather in it somewhere. That prescription that you just picked up at the pharmacy? It probably contains gelatin, and it was almost certainly tested on animals. Latex condoms? They contain milk by-products (seriously!). Will you drink beer? Some beers have isinglass—an ingredient derived from fish swim bladders—in them (see Chapter 4). What about wine? Many wines are clarified with egg products and some wineries even use blood! Unfortunately, in many cases, animal ingredients work their way into thousands of everyday products because as by-products of slaughter, they're inexpensive, plentiful, and easy to obtain.

If you're already sold on ethical veganism, the question becomes one of just how far you can or should reasonably go. Let us be clear: it is reasonable and relatively easy to give up meat, dairy products, eggs, and honey. It is also dead easy to give up leather and wool, and we'll get to those in more depth later. When it comes down to it, we simply don't need those things to live a healthy, happy life, and the only reasons people continue to eat or use them are tradition, preference, and taste. If you notice, these are generally the main reasons meat-eaters throw at you when they want to justify eating meat, and these arguments are not particularly compelling when acute animal suffering is the cost of obtaining these goods (in Chapter 2, we explain why, in depth).

Avoiding the obvious things is usually pretty easy, but what happens when you get beyond the clear-cut issues? You just have to decide for yourself. Though we're not suggesting you consume products

---

5. By ethical vegan, we simply mean a person who has become vegan out of ethical concerns.

of animal exploitation and oppression with abandon, we do think that any reasonable person needs to figure out just how far they're willing to go or are capable of going. In other words, if you're to be truly vegan, should you stop driving, taking medicine, and drinking beer?

Well, that's really up to you.

There's a question of practicality to be considered, though. Any thoughtful ethical vegan will want to avoid animal products to the greatest extent possible, but sometimes, it becomes impossible, unaffordable, or just plain unknowable. This isn't permission to do whatever the hell you please; it just means you shouldn't beat yourself up over the small stuff. For example, you probably need to take some kind of transportation to work, that transportation probably involves tires (e.g. your car or a bus), and many brands of tires contain animal products. Are you not going to drive anymore because of this? Not counting our urban readers for whom such a choice is likely easier and more practical, if you choose to skip driving or commuting for this reason, what are the likely side effects? Might your choosing not to work or not to drive have other more negative effects down the road?

Certainly, if you choose not to drive at all, you might actually be doing the cause of animal rights more harm than good, particularly if you're an activist. Take the example of Eddie Lama who was profiled in the amazing film *The Witness*[6]. In his desire to educate the public about the harms of the fur industry, Lama set up a van full of television screens and speakers that he drove around the streets of New York. Without a doubt, Lama's van (which he calls "FaunaVision") has educated thousands, and likely even made a few people vegan along the way. Had he chosen not to set up FaunaVision because of objections over a relatively small amount of animal products in the tires, he likely would not have gotten the word out so widely and saved so many animals. Along similar lines, pictures of animal exploitation that have been responsible for

---

6. You can get your own copy of this on DVD or VHS from Tribe of Heart (http://www.tribeofheart.org/). While you're there, pick up *Peaceable Kingdom*, too.

changing the treatment of animals never would have seen the light of day were the photographers paralyzed by concerns over gelatin. Or, on a more personal level, maybe you'd not make it to volunteer at the no-kill shelter if you couldn't drive.

The point here is that you can spend a lot of time worrying about tiny infractions, but more often than not, this time would be better spent doing things that have more concrete linkages to ending animal exploitation. It makes sense to avoid all animal products as much as possible. That's something all vegans should want. But if you're being paralyzed by your quest to be the completely, utterly, and totally perfect Mother Theresa of veganism, you're likely not doing yourself or the world as much good as you could be. It is simply a matter of attending to the places where the greatest harms are done, and putting your energies there.

A final note for the vegan police or vegangelicals (who we'll go after again in Chapter 3!): if you're the kind of vegan who enjoys picking on other vegans for not being sufficiently vegan on the above counts, you might think about laying off. As hard-core vegans ourselves, we understand your desire at a certain level. We get the idea that people who are half-hearted or pseudo-vegans muddy the definition of veganism. Anyone who eats cheese and calls themselves a vegan should be politely reminded what "vegan" means. We know this can be problematic and lead to a lot of confusion. But do we really need to be picking on people for drinking a beer that might contain isinglass? Rather than denigrating otherwise decent vegans for tiny infractions of your perceived code of veganism, why not use some of that energy towards leafletting a local campus with materials from Vegan Outreach? We guarantee that the leafletting will be more effective than a high and mighty stance of preaching to the choir.

Speaking of annoying vegans, no one appreciates the drawn-out cries of a new vegan who's jonesin' for a cheese fix or dying to eat ice cream. Yes, when you first switch to veganism, you might miss these things, but there are good substitutes (as we discuss in chapter 4) and ultimately, if you give it some thought, most animal products are pretty nasty (for example, most cheeses contain pus, and eggs are essentially reproductive secretions. Yum!). Regardless of whether you miss these things or not, it is important you not act the martyr for being vegan[7]. Remember, if you're vegan for the right reasons, you're there by your own choice, hopefully after having given your reasons some real thought. By being an ethical vegan, you've decided to take responsibility for your food choices and you've made important mental connections between what's on your plate and its role in needless animal exploitation, suffering, and death. Being vegan is about doing what you know is right, and once you've opened yourself to the ethics in question—once you know, say, that milk production causes animals to be killed—what choice do you reasonably have about being vegan if you're going to live a life that's true to your principles?

Think about it this way: if you're a man, you probably have a lot to gain by being a sexist and upholding the conditions of masculine domination in society. By upholding sexism, you could continue to reap the benefits of your masculinity. Even though many men could gain substantially by upholding sexism, many feminist men stand up against sexism. Why? Because it is wrong, they know it, and they know that even if they gain, they're not helping to make the world one that they'd want to live in, and not fighting the bigger problems in question. Similarly, if you're an ethical vegan, you know you can probably personally gain a great deal by just accepting animal suffering and exploitation. You can eat your [insert desired product of animal torture here] if you can just accept that animals must die to produce it. In the same way that many men comfortably uphold sexism, many meat-eaters make this very decision to accept animal suffering for taste, tradition, and convenience. It might be that both the meat-eater and the sexist imag-

---

7. Thanks again here to Dan Peyser for getting us to think about these issues as they relate to veganism.

ine that things will never change, or that they simply accept that this is the "natural" way of the world. As an ethical vegan, however, you surely know that just accepting the completely disgusting conditions of animal agriculture is wrong. The death, dismemberment, and suffering done in the name of the American palate is a disaster. You know it, and you've decided to do something about it by changing your ways.

You're doing what's right.

That's why it is unhelpful to view veganism as a giant sacrifice on your part. In one sense, sure, you are sacrificing what you could have, just as the anti-sexist male sacrifices something by being opposed to sexism. But you don't deserve martyr points for doing what you know is right and living by your ethics. In this way, veganism isn't a sacrifice; it is the necessary step that you must take if you're to live in a way that's true to your principles. If you run around acting like you're some great saint for eschewing animal products and giving up your beloved cheese, eggs, or milk, then you're putting yourself in a rather precarious position. To return to the example of sexism, imagine for a second how absurd it would sound if the anti-sexist male went around whining about what he's given up to stand up for his principles. "Man, if it weren't for equal rights, I'd probably have beaten out that better-qualified woman for the promotion, but I'm big enough to accept that." Maybe you don't see anything wrong with the underlying sentiment of the previous sentence, but we do.

In the end, if you think you're some kind of saint for being an ethical vegan, you're probably being a bit too immodest. There's no doubt you're doing the right thing by being vegan, but if you've decided to do it, you should commit to it, recognize why you're doing it, and work from there. Doing what's right should never seem like a sacrifice. Moreover, being secure in your veganism is one of the best possible ways to communicate to people that veganism is a choice worth making.

Veganism Can Change Your Life!

We feel like a cheesy 2 AM infomercial when we say that, but veganism does change you as a person, and it changes the way that people relate to you. Unlike the infomercials, we're not offering penis enlargement, weight loss, the newest exercise device, or millionaire potential. Instead, what we're offering—for the low, low price of $12.95! ($17.95 Canadian)—are ideas and advice for smoothing your transition to veganism. This book is largely aimed at helping ethical vegans appreciate and deal with what comes along with the major life change that is veganism.

This book is partial, but then again, all books are. We're two relatively young, relatively radical leftist ethical vegans and our veganism is informed by a critique of animal oppression and speciesism (which we'll get to in the next chapter). Likewise, you can expect our writing to also be informed by these concerns and to downplay others. It isn't that we don't think other reasons for being vegan are important, but others cover these reasons with more grace and experience than we can muster, and where appropriate, we point you to those sources.

Our overall goal is to provide support, advice, and suggestions to those who are newly vegan or thinking about becoming vegan. This guide isn't meant to be comprehensive; instead, it is meant to be an entertaining but useful primer for ethical vegans. We've envisioned this book as a gateway into more reading and research on your part, but we have covered most of the basics here as far as ethical veganism goes. Still, we hope this book will get you moving further into reading and thinking about veganism, and possibly spur you into writing and speaking on these issues as well. In order to facilitate this movement, we've included references at the end of each chapter for any book that we mention, and our crack team of researchers (ummm, okay, the two of us) here at the Vegan Freak home office have also compiled some rather in-depth appendices at the end of the book that detail sources for a variety of vegan products, suggestions for extended reading (both in print and on the Internet), and information on vegan/animal rights groups and online communities. Since anything that deals with the Internet gets stale the moment it is printed, we encourage you to visit the companion website for the book at veganfreak.com for updated appendices, resources, and forums where you can talk with other readers.

The rest of the text is arranged in a few linked chapters. After this, in Chapter 2, we provide a basic ethical framework for understanding animal exploitation and speciesism. We link animal oppression with broader forms of oppression and examine the philosophical and legal arguments that can be used to create a compelling framework for recognizing animal rights. By focusing on factory farming, we also examine animal oppression and explain why veganism is a way to combat this exploitation.

In Chapter 3 we help you stay sane by giving you advice about how to talk to family, friends, co-workers, and others when veganism comes up. You might be surprised by our advice (hint: it doesn't involve telling people to go to hell and mind their own business!). In this chapter, we also discuss some surprising challenges that you might face in dealing with other vegetarians.

Veganism is practiced mostly through food choices, and in Chapter 4, we help you to deal with these choices. In particular, we discuss how to survive in restaurants, we provide tips for the travelin' vegan, and we go into some detail about where animal ingredients hide in average stuff in the grocery store. We also give you some hints about new foods to explore that can help to broaden your vegan palette beyond potato chips, soda, and cheap white bread.

Being vegan doesn't mean that you have to forsake fashion. In Chapter 5, we discuss vegan fashion and cosmetics. We detail what kinds of ingredients cosmetics might contain and we provide some advice for dealing with your old leather, wool, and down, as well as providing sources where you can get durable, high-quality, non-sweatshop kick-ass vegan goods. We also discuss vegan toiletries and what to do about non-vegan condoms.

We close the book in Chapter 6 with a brief wrap-up and discussion of how not to go crazy as a vegan.

~~~~~~

If you're contemplating ethical veganism or you already are an ethical vegan, you've resisted years and years of training in our culture which tells you that animals are ours to experiment on, eat, wear, and abuse at our will. Something in you has told you this logic is deeply wrong, and knowing that, your conscience will likely not rest. In this way, the awareness of animal rights that accompanies veganism is a complex gift that's fraught with both possibility and pitfalls. You've come to see the truth about animal exploitation, and that's extraordinarily powerful. This view provides you with the possibility to move beyond animal oppression in your own life, and to encourage others to do the same. The pitfalls, however, come when you have to confront a culture whose dominant views are almost completely opposite yours when it comes to how animals should be treated. As any sociologist can tell you (and Bob knows, because he is one!), there are always costs to going against the established social order or going against "the way things are." You can be made fun of. You can be marginalized. You can be made to feel stupid, radical, or even insane.

In short, you can be made to feel very much The Vegan Freak. This book will help you love the complex gift of vegan freakdom.

Books and Other Sources Mentioned in This Chapter

- *The Pornography of Meat*. Adams, C. Continuum International Publishing Group. (2003).

- *Animal Liberation*. Singer, P. Avon. (1991).

- *Empty Cages: Facing the Challenge of Animal Rights*. Regan, T. Rowman & Littlefield Publishers, Inc. (2004).

- Dan Peyser's Website can be found at: http://thesmokingvegan.blogspot.com.

- Tribe of Heart (producers of good documentaries on animal rights issues) can be contacted at: http://www.tribeofheart.org

- Vegan Freak Companion Website: http://veganfreak.com

chapter two:
in which we get all AR on you

or vegans, we're some mean motherfuckers. We're murderers. That's right—you heard us. We kill unrepentantly, often boiling, steaming, or stir-frying our victims alive with nary a thought for the freedom we're depriving them or the "pain" we're causing them. Sometimes, we even cut them into small pieces and eat them with garlic—and we enjoy it. We're sick and twisted. We're abusive oppressors without a thought to the plight of the oppressed.

Are we suddenly coming clean about some kind of murder spree? Nah. We're just owning up to the portrait that some meat eaters would like to paint of us.

To meat eaters backed into an intellectual corner, you'd think we vegans were the Hannibal Lecters of the vegetable world. As soon as ethical veganism comes up, omnivores inevitably pull out the line about "plant rights." They reason that if you care so much about the harm brought to animals, you should also care about the harm brought to plants. While many vegans do want to create as light an impact on the earth as possible, this isn't what these omnivores aim to get at through their critique. They want to rip apart your argument for ethical veganism with a thousand tiny blows, because if they can muddy the moral terrain just a little bit and show that your choices are absurd, they can give themselves permission not to think about the challenge you pose as a vegan, implicitly or otherwise.

And so, you'll forever hear gripes over the suffering, exploitation, and death you're causing plants, all while the omnivore happily eats chicken, apparently forgetting that it takes several pounds of grain and other plant products to produce a pound of chicken meat. If the omnivore really cared about plant rights, they'd presumably want to cause the death of as few plants as possible by eating the plants directly rather than cycling them through farm animals whose flesh they later consume. But no matter. It is more fun to annoy the hell out of vegans by calling them murderers.

On top of all of this, the plant rights line ignores some pretty common-sense conclusions. Let's do a quick thought experiment. Let's say that you take a head of broccoli and a pig and stand them side by side. If you take a hot poker and touch the broccoli with it, what happens? Just about nothing. The broccoli burns (which probably doesn't smell too good), but it doesn't scream, it doesn't move away, and it shows no reaction to the poker *because it has no central nervous system or pain receptors*. If, on the other hand, you apply the hot poker to the pig, the pig screams out in pain and runs away. While we can never *truly* know how any other human or non-human being feels, subtle social cues (like screaming) let us make educated guesses about the states of others. Apart from language, the pig reacts much like we would to the hot poker because it *has a central nervous system and pain receptors* much like ours. The plant? Well, let's just say that it's vegetative—literally.

The utter absurdity of the plant rights line shows the extent that people will go to in denying claims of animal suffering. Omnivores, directly or indirectly, are responsible for the bloody death of animals capable of feeling pain, yet they want to come down on vegans for eating broccoli? Yeah, the universe can really be this messed up.

Sadly, this is what we all must face as vegans, particularly if we're ethical vegans. Because of the rampant narcissism of consumer culture, most people will accept your veganism if it's for health reasons. Tell them you're trying to lose a few pounds, or that your cholesterol is high, and they're completely sympathetic to your choices, even if they do see them as extreme. They'll probably even go out of their way to tell you how "brave" you are for suffering through a life without animal foods. If, on the other hand, you tell them you're a vegan because you think animals deserve not to be killed for our enjoyment, you are suddenly slotted away as the vegan freak. The moment you mention animal rights or ethics, most people look at you like you just farted, and they don't know what to say. The most amazing thing is that vegans get this kind of static despite the fact that just about everyone who has a dog or a cat knows animals are capable of feeling pain, experiencing emotions like joy, sadness, and excitement, and have a completely legitimate interest in not suffering. Yet, because of the repressive social machinery we live under and because of our traditions, tastes, and habits, we continue to deprive animals of what they deserve: freedom from pain and exploitation and the ability to live a full life as conscious beings. Rather than thinking critically about the incredible suffering in each bite of meat, dairy, and eggs and how we exploit animals for our own gain and pleasures, we generally think about how much we'd miss Buffalo wings, hamburgers, or cheese[1]. We know we're not the only ones who see this as a disturbing equation.

Working from this basic disconnect between meat and animals in our culture in this chapter we come out all hardcore AR[2] on you. Here we discuss some of the ethical, environmental, and health reasons for going and staying vegan. Our emphasis in this chapter is on the ethical reasons for veganism, working from logical arguments about pain and sentience to contend that exploiting animals for our own ends is mor-

---

1. If you're not yet at this point (say, you're not-quite-vegan), please hang in there. We will offer compelling arguments throughout this chapter as to why you might want to contemplate ethical veganism. You may disagree with us, but at least do us—and the animals—the favor of hearing us out!
2. AR = Animal Rights

ally wrong. We trace some contemporary legal and philosophical thinking on this issue, and argue that we need to more fully develop an appreciation of the rights of animals to live without suffering. Our main argument in this section is that animals are not ours to exploit, and we examine some of the common roots of animal and human oppression (can anyone say CAPITALISM?), how they're tied together, and how fighting for animal rights and human rights aren't mutually exclusive. In addition, we discuss factory farming and why it is an emerging disaster for animals, people, and the environment. We also attack a popular argument used to justify veganism that really annoys us (mostly because it is just plain wrong). In closing the chapter, we examine the health-based arguments for veganism and argue for an ethical and moral practice of animal rights in everyday life.

However, before we start, please indulge us on two important points:

First, though we're also alarmed by circuses, zoos, fisheries, vivisection, hunting, and fur industries, we think the argument against animal agriculture is the most immediately compelling. For one thing, this is the primary way most people are involved in animal exploitation. For another, this is where the overwhelming majority of animal deaths occur. For these reasons, we focus on agriculture at the expense of other animal exploitation industries. Please don't take this to mean that we think fur is fine, or that dissection is good, or that rodeos are fun. We think they all suck, we wish they would stop immediately[3]. Nevertheless, our focus here is largely on agriculture.

Second, a note on the references: in most other chapters, we're pretty loose about how we cite the books that we're using, just putting in a list at the end. Because this chapter depends so much upon references, we've been a bit more careful here, referring to each reference by number in brackets. This'll make it easier for you to track down particular ideas and read up on those in more depth should you so choose.

---

3. If you want to get a good, quick overview of industries of animal exploitation, we heartily recommend *Empty Cages* by Tom Regan.

Okay? Cool. Now, let's talk about Simon the Sadist.

Simon the Sadist

In his book *Introduction to Animal Rights: Your Child or the Dog,* Gary Francione proposes a stunning hypothetical that illustrates the problems with the way we view animals in our culture[1]. To take Francione's hypothetical, imagine there's a nasty bastard named Simon the Sadist who gets off on torturing a dog by burning the dog with a blowtorch. Now, as a non-facetious question, ask yourself: is there anything wrong with this? If you're like us, you can't say "hell yeah!" quickly enough. Anyone with any conscience whatsoever can see that there's plenty wrong with this scenario. As far as we can tell, Simon is subjecting a dog to horrible torture, and it is clear the dog suffers for this torture. It squeals in pain, it recoils, and it pulls away. Were we to ask Simon why he was torturing the dog, his only response would be that he enjoys doing it, and that it gives him great pleasure.

This seems objectionable to most reasonable people. Here's a whack-job who's torturing dogs because he feels like it and enjoys it. Beyond that, he can't really give us any other reason. We're going to venture a guess and say that you don't have to be a vegan to find this deeply problematic. But why do we find it so very problematic? If asked, most people would say the dog feels pain, and would agree that he should not be subjected to undue pain. The dog knows he's being tortured and has every interest in not being tortured. Seems pretty clear, right? In the end, most of us would simply say there's no need for it.

In addition, most people would likely extend this kind of thinking outward to other animals as well. Most folks would say that we shouldn't blowtorch cows or pigs or chickens or anything else either; and when we see these kinds of animal abuse cases, we're usually completely shocked by them. This kind of blatant torture and death feels unnecessary to us, because we understand that at some level animals suffer. Most people—whether vegan or not—would understand these kinds of problems and object to them[4].

If most people can agree these things hold in principle, then how can most people eat meat, dairy, and eggs in practice? If we can agree animals should not face undue suffering for our pleasure, how can we justify killing animals for meat? As many vegans demonstrate, it is completely feasible to live a healthy and vital life without animal products of any kind. Considering we can live quite well without animal products, our consumption of them cannot be chalked up to anything but preference and tradition. And if we truly have an interest in keeping animals free from suffering, our preference for meat is no more valid than Simon's preference for blowtorching animals. Period.

Despite this, somehow we're in a place where we see killing, dismembering, and consuming animals as okay, and blowtorching as "bad." Where we see blowtorching as capricious, we see our desire for the by-products of animal exploitation as "tradition" and "the natural way." Yes, it may be "tradition" to eat meat, but it is also "tradition" in some parts of the country to exclude women from certain jobs, to deny gay people the same rights as straights, and to discriminate against people of color. As for the "natural way" argument, how come we never hear anyone talking of "the natural way" when bears eat infants (as recently happened in New York State), or when crocodiles bite people? Also, what is so "natural" about going to a grocery store and buying a bloody hunk of flesh wrapped in Styrofoam and plastic?

At this point, some of you out there may object to this whole hypothetical by arguing that Simon is in fact torturing animals, while the animals used for our food are not explicitly tortured. True enough, animals are not routinely blowtorched on their way to the average meat eater's plate. Nevertheless, they are, variously, de-beaked, castrated, and de-horned—without the aid of anesthetics—as routine parts of meat,

---

4. As an interesting note, in the real world Simon would be charged with animal abuse, unless he worked in a slaughterhouse, in which case he's "just doing his job." (thanks to Dan Peyser for this observation)

dairy, and egg production. This says nothing of the completely deplorable conditions farm animals live in, often with limited space, light, and fresh air. To take just the example of egg-laying hens, chickens are often crammed into a tiny cage, and not allowed to move outside of that cage until they go to slaughter [2]. Chickens must also have their beaks removed so they do not consume themselves and one another from the psychological stress of their confinement. In addition, male chicks, considered useless to the egg industry, are routinely discarded in dumpsters, suffocated, crushed, or ground up—*alive*. Treatment of living animals aside, don't forget that animals are frequently slaughtered by having their throats slit, while chained by the ankle and hanging upside down. Though part of modern slaughter methods includes incapacitating the animals, this incapacitation is not always effective. In short, contemporary agricultural production practices subject animals to conditions that essentially enslave the animals to our whims. We may not explicitly blowtorch animals in food production, but the other methods used aren't much better. And why? Because people like the taste of eggs, dairy, and meat. There's simply no other reason.

Yes, ovo-lacto vegetarians, you heard us right. We included eggs and dairy there. Some of you borderline vegan folks might imagine (as we once did) that by abstaining from meat, you're abstaining from the death involved in animal agriculture. Unfortunately, this couldn't be further from the truth. The moment dairy cows stop being productive enough or stop being able to get pregnant, they're turned into cheap ground beef and other products. It is important to remember that veal production directly relies on the dairy industry as well. When a cow gives birth to a male, there isn't much dairy farmers can do with them, so they're sold as veal calves. When egg-laying chickens get too old and don't lay enough eggs, they're turned into meat as well. There's no magical pasture where Bessy goes after her "long" life as a milker; there's no special hen house for the older birds. They're simply put to death and eaten. Though it is nice and comforting to imagine otherwise, *by consuming dairy and eggs, you are directly supporting the slaughter of animals* (even if you don't eat the animal yourself). This applies to free range and organic stuff too, so you can't escape that way either. If you believe there's no justification for animal suffering, if you wouldn't see the justification in making another being suffer *simply for your pleasure,* you must consider the impact of dairy and eggs, even if you *really* like eggs and *really* like dairy products.

We say this not to offend borderline- or almost-vegan readers, but to drive home the point that one must truly balance one's desire for the products of animal exploitation with the knowledge that animals are literally tortured and killed for these desires. Gary Francione's hypothetical asks us directly to consider the differences. Just as we can live without torturing animals, we can live without meat, dairy, and eggs. In both cases, there's nothing more pressing than our own desire when it comes down to it. Is our desire for animal products enough to justify the fact that in the time it took you to read this sentence about 500 animals were killed for food[1]? Is it enough to justify the slaughter of more than 8 billion animals a year in the United States alone[1]?

Speciesism

You have to say this: there's something fascinating about a culture that can have such deep moral contradictions. On the one hand, we look at Simon as though he's sick and twisted, and on the other, we consume animals gleefully, with little thought of the miserable conditions they endure. At one level, we can do this because we're at a comfortable distance from the production of our food, so we really don't have to think about the torture involved in getting animal products to our plates. The system that delivers animal products is structured such that we don't have the opportunity to see the vast amounts of suffering it involves. If this suffering was routinely on display, we suspect many, many more people would become vegans—and this is likely why some states are increasing the penalties for shooting unauthorized video in agricultural operations. Nevertheless, we aren't encouraged to think about where our food comes from, and for many of us, that's just fine, thank you very much.

The fact that we're able to condemn Simon and condone meat eating shows the "schizophrenia" we have with regard to animals[1]. We can't decide if we want to love them or eat them, but somehow, we're able to do both. We've compartmentalized animals in our heads. There are "pets" and there are "farm animals" and even though we've not given these divisions much thought, they seem to work well for most people, simply because this is what we've culturally agreed to and grown up with.

The fact that we're able to so conveniently overlook these distinctions makes most of us and our culture *speciesist*. To our knowledge, this term was first coined by Peter Singer in his book *Animal Liberation*[3]. There, Singer defines speciesism as "a prejudice or attitude of bias in favor of the interests of members of one's own species and against those of other species." Speciesism is comparable to other forms of discrimination, particularly racism and sexism, both of which violate principles of equal treatment, and base the unequal treatment on characteristics that are irrelevant. Much as a racist will refuse to hire a Latino simply because he is Latino, a speciesist will justify the exploitation of animals *simply because they are animals*. Driving this point home, Singer writes:

> "Racists violate the principle of equality by giving greater weight to the interests of members of their own race when there is a clash between their interests and the interests of those of another race. Sexists violate the principle of equality by favoring the interests of their own sex. Similarly, speciesists allow the interests of their own species to override the greater interests of members of other species."

This is particularly troubling since animals can be shown to feel fear and pain, be sentient, and suffer tremendously. Given that animals possess the physiological equipment to suffer much like we do, what right do we have to subject them to pain that we ourselves would not want to experience, particularly when that pain is completely unnecessary? The cultural justifications for this torture tend to be nothing but speciesist. Think about it: when people argue that "this is the way it has always been," they're not talking about a logical state of affairs, they're appealing to some abstract sense of tradition. The justifications for consuming animals and animal products tend to weakly fall out along these lines.

For Bob, the links between speciesism and racism really hit home when he started teaching a class on animal rights at the University. After asking students to write about their take on animal rights, many expressed sentiments such as "exploiting animals is in the interests of the human race;" "it is the natural way of the world for one stronger species to dominate another;" "this is the way it has always been;" and "species must show a clear preference for their own kind." Taken together, one could substitute a few words here and there and easily sow this into the propaganda for white supremacists. Granted, the students wrote most of these sentiments before they had a chance to consider Singer and other animal rights theorists, powerfully illustrating the currency these ideas have in our culture.

It is important to note here that speciesism is part of the greater problem of exploitation of both human and non-human animals. In any kind of baseless discrimination, there is necessarily a common form of "othering" going on in which the person being discriminated against is considered to be *less than* the person who's doing the discriminating. The racist assumes the person of color is *less than* he is; the sexist assumes the woman is *less than* the man; the homophobe assumes the gay person is *less than* the straight. A speciesist assumes that animals are *less than* humans, and so their exploitation is justified. This common process at the root of all discrimination—be it human or non-human—cannot be ignored if we're to understand how discrimination is built into the very structure of our society and culture.

Domination and oppression of humans and other animals is enabled by economic exploitation, unequal power, and ideological control[4]. Much as slave holders in the south happily exploited slaves when it was in their interest to do so, most human cultures will happily exploit animals for profit. Unequal power aids exploitation, mostly because the routes of fighting back are limited. Finally, ideological control convinces us that exploitation and oppression are natural and in our interest, making the oppression largely invisible. This dynamic explains how oppression is built into the very fabric of our day-to-day lives and social order.

At one level, trying to explain animal cruelty to people who happily consume animal products is like trying to explain water to the fish. Even though few people can put forth any reasonable justification for the deaths of so very many animals, many people still view consuming animals as the natural and normal state of affairs because they've grown up in a culture where this exploitation is accepted and commonly taught. As an ethical vegan, you face the challenge of confronting this culture of oppression just about everyday, and it can be frustrating. You probably often wonder why everyone can't just see the world as you see it, why they can't see the obvious suffering involved in things we consume every single day. Often, instead of being praised for your ability to think independently and move beyond your social training, you're left out in the cold. Making you feel like the freak is part of the way that our culture continues to keep speciesism alive. Being tagged this way is the social price you're paying for going against the established order, and this is why so many people think vegans are freaks.

Freakdom aside, it is important to keep in mind the ways in which various forms of oppression are linked and inseparable. In *The Dreaded Comparison*[5], Marjorie Spiegel talks about how animal slavery and human slavery are linked, sometimes with harrowing illustrations. Similarly, in *Eternal Treblinka: Our Treatment of Animals and the Holocaust*[6], Charles Patterson examines the history of eugenics in America, how it was linked to animal husbandry, and how the Nazis picked up on these practices to drive the extermination of Jews and others in the Holocaust. Comparing pornography and the treatment of women in her book *The Pornography of Meat*[7], Carol Adams shows how exploitation of women and animals is justified in similar ways. In considering these books, a portrait of the ways that speciesism is linked to other forms of discrimination emerges. Though the books themselves are sometimes very difficult reads for the potency of the ideas they express, they are powerful reminders that sexism, racism, and speciesism do not stand independent of one another as forms of social oppression. We recommend all of these texts, as they'll give you plenty to think about.

Along these lines, when you speak to friends about animal rights, you're likely to hear that we should be "paying attention to people first." If you've been an ethical vegan for any time at all, you've probably already heard people tell you they'll happily solve the problems of animal exploitation just as soon as we get to solving all of the problems of human exploitation. Sadly, meat-loving leftists are often the first to come out with this ultimately weak argument, and also sadly, as Peter Singer points out, they're usually not doing a damn thing for people *or* animals. Quite predictably, our response to these people tends to highlight the idea that all forms of oppression are linked. Working to end one form of oppression necessarily helps to illustrate other forms of oppression. Put even more simply, who ever said that working for human rights and animal rights are mutually exclusive ends? Many animal rights activists are also committed to other areas of social justice, and seeing animal rights as outside of other social justice causes is just plain shortsighted.

Speciesism and Capitalism

Considering all of this, it should be clear by now that speciesism is how we justify the horrific uses that animals are put to in our culture; it is the mental framework we've constructed over time to give ourselves the freedom to do as we please with animals. When this inherent bias towards animals is coupled with our current economic system, the results are disastrous for the animals, the environment, and our health. And to think, you probably always learned that capitalism was A Very Good Thing!

If you grew up during the Reagan years like we did, you surely remember being afraid of getting nuked by those nasty commies, and you probably also remember learning that American-style free market capitalism was the solution to all the world's problems. This has morphed into an operating assumption today that free markets bring free minds and democracy[5]. Government regulation is also seen as A Very Bad Thing. Coupled together with capitalism's inherent and insatiable desire for profit, the decline in regulation and government intervention in business has meant that in many spheres, economic interests trump all others—health, the environment, and rights be damned. Though our current capitalist economic system can provide a few of us with a pretty good standard of living, the question is, upon whose backs is that standard of living built?

Under capitalism, we're able to eat like only royalty could in the past (which we'll discuss in depth later in this chapter). If you live in a Western country, you can literally have meat, dairy, and eggs for every meal for every day of your life, and you really don't have to be all that rich to have them. To the people who think Crisco is something you spread on crackers[6] this is completely freakin' awesome. To the people and animals who are exploited to bring us this kingly banquet, things don't look quite so hot. And it is here, at this intersection between living—pardon the pun—high on the hog and getting screwed over that we begin our discussion of how the economic system we all live under helps to intensify animal suffering to a shocking degree.

Think about the things we consume. We rarely—if ever—see the producers and the process of production that go into the million goods that we buy. Instead, we walk into a shop, plunk down our hard-earned cash, and walk out with wicked cool stuff (technical economic term, that is). Though we do this just about every single day, there's a lot hidden in this seemingly basic process. We don't see who produced what we've bought, we don't see the conditions they labored in to produce it, and we don't see the impact of the resources extracted to make the product. In a sense, products just appear on store shelves "as if by magic." Conveniently, this is the way those who have the most to gain prefer

---

5. How come everyone always forgets about China being a (largely) free market country when they say this?
6. Check the Crisco label: they tell you not to do this!

that we see it. Why get all bothered by the idea that someone might have been exploited to produce your steak when you can just buy the steak, go home, eat it, and sleep peacefully in blissful ignorance? And if you had to think about the gory backstory, would you really buy so much steak?

As consumers, we're separated from producers and the way things are produced. Karl Marx called this the "commodity fetish." He didn't mean that we got all hot and crazy over stuff; instead, he meant that we tended to see the things we buy as only *things*, instead of seeing all of the labor and other factors involved in the production of these things. Because of this basic dynamic of capitalism, many of us can guiltlessly consume whatever we please, be it steak, clothes, or iPods. In addition, those who invest in production also want to see the greatest possible return on their investment. When you put this together with the fact that most of us don't even remotely care about where the stuff we buy comes from, you can see the stage being set for some pretty funky (bad funky, not good funky) business. Corporations have their products made in the places with the lowest possible wages; call centers are "outsourced;" and just about everything is made in China these days.

When we take these dynamics and apply them to animal agriculture, a shocking portrait emerges. Three things come together to make life hell for animals involved in food production: first, speciesism justifies not only the consumption of animals as "lesser" creatures, but also allows us to do just about anything we wish to them; second, the desire to make the most profit means that animals are viewed as "economic units," and their "profit potential" is maximized as much as possible, which often leads to excessively cruel treatment; and third, we don't think about where our products come from, which makes it easy for those raising farm animals to do practically whatever they please—without questions from the consumers—in pursuit of more profit. When we take these things together in an era of decreasing regulation, it becomes easy to see how factory farming has emerged as a force to be reckoned with in America.

Factory Farming and Animal Exploitation

If you pick up enough children's books, sooner or later you're bound to come across one about farm animals. These books almost always display the lives of farm animals as peaceful romps across sunny pastures, and somehow, we never end up advancing much beyond this storybook view of the way animals are raised.

A simple rule Bob learned in college about today's agriculture is that in order to be profitable, you have to be big. If you want to make any money at all, really, you have to have not just 100 or 200 cattle, but thousands. Similarly, because profit margins are so slim, you need to raise animals in the cheapest possible way, and part of doing this comes from routinizing every single aspect of the life of a farm animal, from birth to slaughter and beyond. In the case of cows, this has meant moving animals away from pasture and into feedlots, where they're literally jammed cheek to jowl. In addition, animals are often loaded up with antibiotics to fight infections that can easily get out of hand in such intensive confinement. For chickens, there's no scratching around in the soil and eating bugs; instead, most chickens now live their entire lives inside a single cage—with 6 other birds—in a single building. Current agricultural methods, at least as practiced by the largest, most profitable, and most productive firms, contrast drastically with the agriculture of only 50 years ago, which was a bit closer in practice to what you see in those children's books. Though animals also suffered slaughter 50 years ago, they generally had a better quality of life than animals today who rarely see pasture, get fresh air, or enjoy much freedom of movement. This kind of agriculture that considers animals as mere "inputs" in an economic process is actually the state-of-the-art for agricultural education—and Bob knows, because he learned many of these methods. In his book *Mad Cowboy*[8], Howard Lyman talks about his own experience in agricultural education, how he applied what he learned in college to his own farm, and how he eventually came to see this as a loss of what was good about agriculture.

Though it is beyond the scope of this book to provide a detailed account of the processes of factory farming, we will provide a quick overview of some of the practices grouped by animal and commodity to give you a sense of what goes on. If you're after more detail, we'd encourage you to check out Erik Marcus's latest book *Meat Market: Animals, Ethics, and Money*[2], as well as Tom Regan's *Empty Cages: Facing the Challenge of Animal Rights*[9]. Both of these texts can provide you with many more harrowing details than we can share in the short space available to us here. In particular, Marcus provides a sweeping overview of the economics of animal agriculture, the wrongs involved in animal production, and what we can do to fight animal exploitation in agriculture.

Eggs and Chicken

In a talk that Erik Marcus gave at our University, he made the point that pound for pound, the most suffering is found in chicken and eggs. In *Meat Market* he gives plenty of reasons why he sees this as the case. Egg-laying hens face a life that is unthinkably cruel. From almost the moment they are born, layer chicks are subjected to unimaginable cruelty. Because males are unprofitable, they're often ground up alive, or simply discarded to starve[7]. Females are separated out and have their beaks seared off by a hot blade in a machine. This is necessary because when the birds are later crammed into confinement for egg production, they would otherwise peck one another to death. Hens are put into cages so small, they cannot even spread their wings. For two years, they will labor in these conditions, each hen having less space to live in than your average letter-sized piece of paper, producing eggs. They are also occasionally forced to molt to increase their productivity by being starved for up to two weeks with the lights on 24/7. After these chickens have reached the end of their productive lives, they're slaughtered. If you think this sounds extreme, we would encourage you to have a look at the investigations by Compassion Over Killing (http://www.

---

7. Come on, on the fence almost vegans! How can this *not* convince you to give up eggs?!

cok.net/camp/inv/egg.php) that show that what Marcus describes is the *standard* treatment. Often, animals end up in much worse conditions.

Layer hens have a somewhat different life than your average broiler chicken. The average chicken house for broiler chickens now "holds upwards of 20,000 chickens with each bird getting less than a square foot of space"[2]. Meat chickens are similarly caged, but killed after only seven weeks of growth.

Pigs

We all have something in our pasts that we regret, and Bob is going to share something out of his that bothers him to this day. For part of a college internship, long before Bob was a vegetarian or vegan, he had to work for a few days on a pig farm in Ohio. Without a doubt, this is one of the experiences that got Bob seriously thinking about vegetarianism, and though he's now ashamed to admit that he took part in this cruelty, he thinks it is worth recounting his experience here to give you a sense of what piglets go through.

While working on the pig farm, one of Bob's jobs was to prepare baby male piglets for their lives (and deaths) as meat animals. This work involved castrating the piglets, clipping their teeth, and notching their ears so they could be identified correctly. Picking up each piglet, Bob would flip them over, quickly swab their lower belly with disinfectant, and then make two small incisions with a blade to remove the testicles. This was all done without benefit of anesthetic, and the piglets screamed horribly; even as an omnivore, Bob could only do a few of these castrations before refusing to do more. In addition to castration, the piglets' ears were notched with a tool that literally cut out sections of the ear (again, without anesthetic) several times to indicate their identity. Both of these procedures were done at the same time, subjecting the piglets to significant pain.

In addition to the things Bob himself witnessed, the tails of pigs are cut off so that they avoid biting one another in overcrowded conditions[2]. After this, pigs are kept for four months in a "finishing shed" where they're fed until they get to about 260 pounds, at which point they're transported to slaughter[2].

Dairy Cattle and Veal

The free-roaming dairy cattle that we imagine as the norm are increasingly a thing of the past. As it becomes more cost efficient to feed animals set feed mixtures[8], cows are kept in what are called dry-lot operations, either fenced in to a small space outdoors, or kept in a metal-roofed shed[9]. In order for cows to give the approximately 2000 gallons of milk they produce annually, they must be pregnant, and they are kept pregnant for nine months out of every year. When the cows give birth, the calves are separated from their mothers within 48 hours; farmers keep the milk, and the calves get formula. The female calves are then turned into dairy cows, and the males are often sold as veal calves. Unproductive or under-productive cows are sent to slaughter.

When one stops to consider the direct linkages between the dairy industry and the slaughter of animals, it becomes hard to ignore that dairy consumption is supporting the death of animals. Old dairy cows are often turned into beef, and the male calves of dairy cows become veal. Commenting on this, Erik Marcus writes "Activists often say that each glass of milk contains a bit of veal, and in a sense, this is true."[2]

Meat Sucks for People Too

While it is obvious animals don't fare well at slaughter, neither do workers in the slaughterhouses. The horrible conditions slaughterhouse workers face is yet another aspect of meat production we're happy to ignore. Earlier, we cited the figure of 8 billion animals slaughtered annually in the United States. Someone has to be doing all of this rapid killing. Modern slaughterhouses move very fast to accommodate the large numbers of animal carcasses that must be turned into meat. In *Fast Food Nation*[10], Eric Schlosser details some of the conditions

---

8. Including, possibly, other ground up animals of the same species, increasing the risk for mad cow and similar diseases.
9. Unless otherwise noted, all figures in this section are from *Meat Market*.

slaughterhouse workers must endure, including the risks of severely cutting oneself and repetitive stress injuries. Because many illegal immigrants work in slaughterhouses, they often do not even seek worker's compensation benefits for fear of being caught. Echoing Schlosser's book, Human Rights Watch has written that the slaughter industry sees "extraordinarily high rates of injury" and systematically violates *human* rights[11].

Factory Farming and the Environment

Not only does factory farming lead to the torture of animals and exploitation of labor, it is also wreaking havoc on the environment. In an effort to avoid regulation, maximize profits, and keep costs down, agribusiness has poisoned our water and air, helped push global warming further along, destroyed wildlife, fragile habitats and ecosystems, and monopolized valuable land and water supplies that could be going toward much better uses.

One of the most common statistics you hear in connection with factory farming is that it takes 16 pounds of grain to make one pound of beef, because it demonstrates how wasteful the process is. Yes, that 16 pounds of grain could be going directly to feed people (more on that later), but the lack of efficiency isn't the only waste; it takes untold amounts of water, fossil fuel, and chemicals to create that beef. Large-scale animal farms in the Midwest are rapidly depleting what is called the Ogallala aquifer, a vast supply of underground water which has been accumulating for hundreds of thousands of years[12], because 70% of the water in the Western states goes toward animal agriculture[8]. All intensive agriculture is dependent on fossil fuels, but animal agriculture even more so because of that 16 to 1 ratio. It takes approximately 140 gallons of oil to produce one acre of grain, since petroleum is used to create the pesticides and herbicides, as well as to run the farm machinery[12]. Another way to view this statistic, taking into account the transportation of cattle as well, is that it takes 260 gallons of fossil fuel to provide beef for a family of 4 for a year, in the process releasing 2.5 tons of carbon dioxide into the atmosphere[13].

The extra carbon dioxide—the greenhouse gas which is the largest contributor to global warming—isn't the only pollution that comes from factory farms. Cattle produce methane—the second-largest greenhouse gas—at the rate of 150 trillion quarts per year [8]. In addition, our water supply is being polluted not only by pesticides and herbicides from the grain crops, but also by the dumping of manure. As a result, our water has high levels of ammonia, nitrates, bacteria, and other microscopic organisms, which not only kill fish and other aquatic life, but also represent a significant danger to human health[8]. And manure doesn't just pollute the water—it can pollute the air. In November 2004, a 2000-ton pile of manure at a feed lot caught fire in Nebraska, and they couldn't put it out for over three months[14]. Overall, the air and water pollution isn't just from raising meat; this pollution is also from dairy farms, as well as chicken and egg farms that deposit amazing amounts of manure into the water supply.

As if the air and water pollution weren't enough, intensive animal agriculture is destroying our land and the wildlife that used to dwell there. The herds of cattle that graze in the Midwest contribute to soil erosion by depleting the grasses. In addition, the action of the hooves of so many large animals[8] also contributes to soil erosion. This destroys the land in the west by causing desertification, depleting the natural landscape and turning it into non-viable land. In addition, to protect these "valuable commodities" of livestock (AKA living beings), ranchers kill prairie dogs, birds, coyotes, large cats, foxes, wolves, and bears that might prey on the cattle or harm them otherwise [12].

The lust for beef doesn't just destroy landscapes and habitats in North America; rain forests in countries like Brazil are being cut down to make way for cattle farms and ranches, so that the meat can be sold to the US and other first world countries. For this reason, veganism is linked to questions of hunger in the developing world. In the next section, we tackle what we see as the accurate arguments for veganism and the alleviation of hunger and also take on what we see as problematic approaches to dealing with these issues.

Veganism and Hunger: Truth and Fiction

There are two kinds of arguments about veganism and its effects on hunger—one accurate, the other a bit mistaken. Let's get at the more accurate argument first.

Given the global nature of agricultural production, some people argue that animal agriculture leads to the destruction of native ecosystems in the developing world as countries clear forests for grazing and other kinds of animal agriculture. The meat produced this way is often shipped to the developed world, so it isn't even helping to address hunger problems at its source. On top of this, all of the land dedicated to animal agriculture means that subsistence-based farmers have less land to grow food for themselves and their families. People starve as they export food[10]. This basic dynamic, at least in the broad outlines, is correct, so we'd say that this is the solid argument, if only in the sense that were demand for meat to decrease, we might see this dynamic be less pronounced.

The second kind of argument you'll hear about veganism and hunger goes like this: if we stopped feeding grain to animals to turn it into meat, we'd free up grain we could directly feed to people. Peter Singer himself argues this very point in *Animal Liberation:*

"Those who claim to care about the well-being of human beings and the preservation of our environment should become vegetarians for that reason alone. They would thereby increase the amount of grain available to feed people elsewhere, reduce pollution, save water and energy, and cease contributing to the clearing of forests."[3]

Though there are valid arguments for veganism's link with reducing environmental harm, this argument that ties veganism to hunger is just plain wrong, and we wish people would stop using it. In principle, it is

---

10. During a famine in the 1980s, Ethiopia was actually exporting food to Europe, showing just how strong this dynamic actually is.

a noble sentiment: hey, if we just stop feeding all that grain to animals, we can give it to people, right?

Ummm, no.

The problem that we face in hunger isn't an issue of food scarcity. On the whole, there is more than enough food production worldwide to feed everyone. Unfortunately for those who don't have enough to eat, the problem of hunger is more complex than this simple argument assumes. Global hunger is a political, economic, and social phenomenon, and simply having more food available doesn't mean fewer people will starve. If those who are hungry cannot gain access to land to grow their own crops or afford to buy food, they will perish even if there is grain rotting away in storage (as has been the case for many years). The main problem of hunger is a question of *distribution* of existing food supplies and who controls that distribution. Because the global agricultural market is about making money (and foreign aid is about politics) the question of who gets to eat and who doesn't will always be influenced by these economic and socio-political questions. Even if every vegan freed up several tons of grain every single day by not eating meat, it wouldn't make even the tiniest dent in global hunger. In all honesty, the grain would probably go moldy or be destroyed to keep prices up before it was given away to feed the hungry of the world.

Though the world is set up this way, don't take this to mean we like it. Keeping people from what they need to live is a form of violence. It bothers us that Americans are literally dying of diseases of *overconsumption* while 800 or so million people in the world are hungry[15]. We just get frustrated when we hear vegans make this argument because it ignores the real and complex reasons for global hunger. Veganism is the solution to a great many problems, but hunger has to be attacked differently, likely by targeting the global capitalist economy—which is the subject of another set of books entirely. So, if you find yourself trying to use this argument against meat eaters, you might think twice about it. It is a nice wish for the way the world *could be* but it has little merit in fact.

~~~~~~

Up to this point, we've discussed the question of animal rights and speciesism, and the ways animal agriculture abuses animals and harms the environment. Veganism offers a compelling solution to avoiding many of these problems. Besides being a way to minimize animal exploitation and environmental degradation, veganism can be extraordinarily healthy if done wisely. In the next section, we discuss some of the health benefits of veganism, touching on vegan nutrition and its relation to diet. You'll see veganism makes sense not only for animals, but also for your own health.

Vegan Health or "Oh my God if you don't eat animal protein you will die a horrible and ugly death."

Let us just state outright and up front that you do not need to ingest any animal products to be healthy. If you're not vegan yet, maybe you haven't made the switch because somewhere in the back of your mind you think that milk and eggs give you nutrients that you absolutely need, or you're thinking about that story an ex-vegetarian told you about not getting enough iron. Or maybe you just think vegetarians are just as healthy as vegans.

Many people have the misconception that the vegan diet is unhealthy, most likely because they see it as somehow deficient (where do you get your protein?) or, as we describe in Chapter 3, they see it as a form of deprivation in comparison to their normal diet. In addition, Western society has made us think we need meat and milk in order to be healthy, partially in an attempt to imitate a lifestyle that in the past only the wealthy could have, and mostly to fill the coffers of the dairy and meat industries and lobbies. Thanks to years upon years of meat and dairy council direct marketing to nutritionists, schools, and others, these ideas have become deeply ingrained in individuals, and the notion that any alternative is possible is rarely heeded. Some people out there might have the sense that a vegan diet is healthy, but see it as a completely unattainable goal because they see it as too hard, too limiting, and too freaky to be worth any possible gains.

One of the common arguments against a vegan diet is that humans have always been eating the way we eat today (in Western countries), so a vegan diet is "unnatural." A study of history, however, shows that Westerners have only begun to eat a diet heavy in meat and dairy in the last century, following the industrial revolution[16]. In the US and other developed nations, the consumption of meat and dairy has increased even more dramatically since the 1950s, coinciding with the advent of factory farming and other intensive agricultural practices[8]. Before the industrial revolution, only the wealthy—usually nobility of some sort—were able to eat animal foods on a regular basis, while everyone else relied on a plant-based diet and the occasional bit of meat or dairy product. This has been the case since the advent of agriculture approximately 10,000 years ago[16].

The nobility of yesteryear and the person eating the Standard American Diet (SAD) in today's Western society have something in common—they both suffer from what are known as diseases of affluence. These diseases—which include cancer (especially breast, prostate, pancreas, colon), obesity[11], heart disease, hypertension (high blood pressure), high cholesterol, osteoporosis, diabetes, kidney stones and kidney failure, macular degeneration, arthritis, multiple sclerosis and other auto-immune diseases like lupus, and more—are only found in populations that eat meat and dairy at the rate found in the SAD[16, 18]. Today's societies that rely on a plant-based diet have very few occurrences of these diseases[18].

We have come to see these diseases as the norm in our society, but there is an easy way to eliminate them. Doctors and researchers have shown that a whole foods, plant-based diet (this means no dairy or eggs either) can prevent these diseases of affluence, and can also reverse the diseases if they have already begun[18]. This diet is so effective for sev-

---

11. The United States is now the most obese country on the planet[17]. Approximately 1/3 of all adults are obese, and the number is growing fast[18].

eral reasons: it is high in fiber, low in fat and protein, full of vitamins and minerals in their natural state (found to be more effective than supplements, especially for antioxidants), and is cholesterol-free [18]. The vegan diet focused on whole foods, therefore, is arguably the most healthy diet on the planet.

The diet that has sustained humans for centuries is optimally 10% protein, 10% fat, and 80% carbohydrates, nearly all from plant sources[18]. Contrary to the claims of high-protein, low-carb diet fans, not all carbohydrates are bad for you. Carbohydrates, in their unprocessed forms, add fiber and essential nutrients to our diet[12]. In addition, they are the primary source of fuel for our body, especially the brain. Dr. Michael Greger explains in his book *Carbophobia* that when a body isn't able to use carbohydrates as a fuel, it thinks it is starving[17]. By having to rely on fat and protein as a fuel (as in a high-protein diet), the body produces chemicals known as ketones as a by-product, which are toxic and must be excreted through the lungs and kidneys[13] (a state known as ketosis). Because the normal by-products of carbohydrate metabolism are not available, the body has no source of fuel to run correctly and thus no energy. Some of the side effects of this ketosis include bad breath, fatigue, weakness, headaches and dizziness, depression, nausea, and vomiting, not to mention the constipation, muscle cramps, and lack of sex drive from the diet.

The benefits of a high-carbohydrate, low-fat, plant-based diet have been demonstrated in a number of different types of studies, including laboratory experiments, the analysis of the effects of specific diets (like the near-vegan Ornish diet), and long-term observations of the connections between disease and diet. Nutritional biochemist Dr. T. Colin Campbell did long-term studies of the diets of various populations in

---

12. Animal products contain no fiber. Processed carbs like sugar, white flour, and white rice aren't as nutritious since they don't have much fiber and can increase blood sugar and triglyceride levels. Complex carbohydrates in their unprocessed forms lower cholesterol and blood sugar[19].

13. This is why people on high-protein diets initially lose weight - the body uses lots of water to flush out the ketones and you pee it all out.[17]

China, and he sums up the results of these and other nutrition studies in his book *The China Study: Startling Implications for Diet, Weight Loss, and Long-Term Health*[18]. In short, the book describes how animal foods cause all of the diseases of affluence listed above. As you would expect, the fat and cholesterol in the SAD lead to higher rates of heart disease, and the lack of fiber can lead to problems with the colon. In addition, antioxidants are rare in animal foods; the lack of these hinders the body's ability to fight off disease. But one of the most surprising findings in this study is that animal protein is not good for you either. Campbell explains that animal protein acts as a trigger that allows the development of cancer to progress, while plant protein does not. What is more, the protein in milk (casein) is especially dangerous—it has not only been linked to cancer, but also to Type I diabetes and other auto-immune diseases. Therefore, the vegetarian diet is not as effective as the vegan diet in preventing the diseases of affluence, even if you use skim milk and cholesterol-reduced eggs[14].

There are many common misconceptions about the vegan diet, and chances are at some point someone will ask you, "where do you get your protein/calcium/iron?" The basic answer is that a well-balanced vegan diet contains plenty of these nutrients, and in forms that are healthier than animal-based foods because they are easily absorbed and don't come attached to all the fat found in animal products. Foods like broccoli, leafy greens, legumes, tofu and soymilk, grains, figs, and tahini are high in calcium; tofu, beans, spinach, cabbage, wheat germ, whole grains, parsley, figs, dates, apricots, and molasses are good sources of iron; and beans, legumes, tofu, soymilk, whole grains, and tahini will give you all the protein you need[19]. Your body doesn't need tons of protein (i.e. no more than 10%-15% of calories) to be healthy. In addition, eating lower protein levels will help your body retain more of the

---

14. Hear that, ovo-lacto vegetarians? Plus, eggs are just plain unhealthy. They are cholesterol and saturated fat bombs.

calcium that it does get, as extra protein turns the blood more acidic, causing the body to leach calcium out of the bones[19].

And even though we said in the introduction that this book wasn't going to be a treatise on the B12 debate, we do have to mention it here because it might come up in an argument about veganism. At some point, you're apt to hear the plaintive cry that "if humans were supposed to be vegan, then why do they have to take B12 supplements?" All animals have bacteria in their digestive system that produce B12, but humans can't absorb it very well. Omnivores get their B12 through eating other animals. In the past, we could also get B12 from plant sources because bacteria in the soil can also produce B12. As a result, eating produce that came from healthy soil would give you the nutrient[20]. Today's agricultural practices, however, have basically killed the soil with chemicals—it isn't healthy enough to sustain the microorganisms that would produce B12—and all produce is cleaned thoroughly of soil residue. Therefore, it is wise (especially if you don't use enriched soymilk or cereals) to take a supplement every now and then [20].

So, all the evidence shows that you don't need to eat meat, dairy, or eggs to be heathy. Vegans have extremely low incidences of all of the diseases of affluence, at rates lower than vegetarians and much lower than meat-eaters. In fact, a vegan diet will help you live a longer and healthier life, if you eat a whole foods, balanced diet[21]. It is really easy, however, to fall into the trap of the junk-food vegan. You know the one—the vegan who only eats potato chips, fake meats, and soda. And while we are junk food fans ourselves (and love a good meat analog), it's a good idea to remember to vary your diet and eat some fresh veggies once in awhile. Junk food vegans can have some of the problems that vegetarians and meat-eaters have because their diet is also high in fat (which can trigger high cholesterol) and refined carbohydrates. If you're stuck in a food rut, see Chapter 4 for some suggestions on new foods to try, and consult one of the many cookbooks in Appendix B for help as well.

If you're interested in learning more about vegan nutrition, please check out one of the references used in this section—we're not nutritionists (nor do we play nutritionists on TV), we've just read a lot about vegan nutrition. Even if you're primarily an ethical vegan, these books are informative, well-researched, and interesting reads because they do a very good job at providing solid evidence that the vegan diet is the way to go, and at debunking dietary myths ingrained in our society. They are also good inspiration for eating a little healthier than you might be right now.

One more note about nutrition before we move on: as you listen to or read the occasional story about nutrition that comes across the news, learn to take it with a grain of salt. Agribusiness is a huge industry, and they don't take threats to their livelihood lightly. They use their pull with the government to keep the truth about how bad meat, dairy, and eggs are for you out of the press, and to fund studies that will help support their position. Just this year the Centers for Disease Control and Prevention came out with a report stating obesity wasn't so bad for you and might help you live longer, a statement that most people recognized as so over the top that they later had to soften their original reading of the study. In addition, the pharmaceutical industry is quite happy to see people spending billions trying to cure heart disease and cancer with their medicines, so they are not going to appreciate doctors saying that the best way to deal with these problems is prevention through diet. Think we're being paranoid? Then read *The China Study* to hear about it from someone who has experienced the ties between government and industry fist hand.

Veganism is the right choice for animals, your health, and the environment. As the sources above show, you can thrive on a vegan diet. And if you don't have to consume animal products to live a full, healthy, and happy life, are you really any better off morally than our example of Simon the Sadist if you continue to consume them?

In closing this chapter on animal exploitation and veganism, we return to where we started. Arguing for the necessity of animal rights, we consider how veganism is a direct expression of a moral and ethical stance that values animal liberation and rejects animal exploitation. In addition, we argue that your veganism is a powerful reminder that all is not right when it comes to animal exploitation. We can find great joy knowing that our choices bring us closer to an emancipated world for animals and humans alike.

Fighting Animal Exploitation[15]

After everything we've detailed in this chapter, it should go without saying that animal exploitation is horrendous and unnecessary. As sentient beings, animals deserve nothing less than the ability to live their lives free of pain and exploitation. Animals should be treated as beings rather than *things,* and we do not have the inherent right to subjugate other beings for our own purposes. In human society we call that slavery, and when we do it to animals it is no different. There is no "humane" slavery, and just as there is no humane slavery, there can be no "humane" slaughter, exploitation, or abuse of animals. The very act of subjugating animals for our own use is morally objectionable since it denies another being the ability to live its life free of pain and suffering. Sadly, what is often called "animal welfare" consists of minor improvements in the process of subjugating animals. If you're a slave and you live in a bigger room, aren't you still a slave? For this reason, Tom Regan writes that we should not want bigger cages; instead, we should want nothing less than *empty* cages.[9]

Some people object to the idea of animal rights because animals are "irrational" or because they can't speak, yet we give rights to very young children who are also "irrational" and who cannot speak. Being able to speak, or being able to reciprocate rights are not reasons to deny those

---

15. Given the limitations of a book this broadly-based, it is beyond the scope of our work to put forth an in-depth theory of animal rights. If you want that, you should read Francione, Regan, and Singer, all of whom put forth compelling philosophical and moral arguments about animal rights.

rights to anyone, human or non-human. Giving animals rights does not mean that animals are exactly like humans; instead, it means we accept that animals—as sentient possessors of their own lives—deserve to be treated with respect, and deserve to be free from exploitation and oppression. Recognizing animals' rights imposes a moral obligation on us as humans to protect and recognize the interests of animals, and to defer to those interests even when they clash with our own. Such rights could easily be written into law[16], were the impetus to exist. Until then, it is up to those of us who understand that animals are deserving of our respect to remind others of this simple fact.

What's mind-boggling about all of this needless animal exploitation is that the solution is exceedingly simple. Humans can live well as vegans, and there are millions of vegans around the world who prove this to be the case, day in and day out. As ethical vegans, we live as practicing anti-speciesists in a world that exploits animals at every turn. We ethical vegans serve as a constant reminder that something is not right with the use and exploitation of animals, and in this sense, our very diet is a form of living protest we enact at every meal. Veganism is our lived expression of our own ethics; it is basic compassion 101.

Despite this, as a way of easing their own conscience and justifying their own inaction, you'll hear omnivores sincerely tell you that "one person can't change anything." It may be true that you alone will never stop dairy production, or cause the downfall of the egg industry. Still, being vegan is an essential step for anyone who believes in animal rights. It is the most basic commitment anyone can make towards showing that animals are not ours to use and abuse. In addition, part of fighting against speciesism requires that we speak out for those who cannot speak. Though many of us who care about the rights of animals are marginalized by a media that would sooner paint us as "terrorists" than air a documentary on the abuses of animal agriculture, we can have a powerful influence on those around us. We can educate our friends, family, and communities, and show them what's wrong with the way we

---

16. Some of these rights have already been written into law for companion animals.

treat animals. When people who know us see our sincerity on this issue, it can make them rethink their own participation in animal suffering.

If you're not an ethical vegan already, we hope you'll educate yourself further on these issues using the sources in this chapter. There is plenty in those books to consider, mull over, and think about, and our hope is that they will convince you to go vegan and stay vegan.

If, however, you have already made a choice to become vegan, this raises the question of how you remain sane in a world that is so very speciesist and un-vegan. In the next chapter, we provide some advice on how to live out your ethical choices, particularly among family and friends who may or may not be completely cool with your choices.

Books and Other Sources Mentioned in This Chapter

1. *Introduction to Animal Rights: Your Child or the Dog?* Francione, G. Temple University Press. (2000).

2. *Meat Market: Animals, Ethics, and Money.* Marcus, E. Brio Press. (2005).

3. *Animal Liberation.* Singer, P. Avon. (1991).

4. *Animal Rights/Human Rights.* Nibert, D. Rowman & Littlefield Publishers. (2002).

5. *The Dreaded Comparison: Human and Animal Slavery.* Spiegel, M. Mirror Books. (1996).

6. *Eternal Treblinka: Our Treatment of Animals and the Holocaust.* Patterson, C. Lantern Books. (2002).

7. *The Pornography of Meat.* Adams, C. Continuum International Publishing Group. (2003).

8. *Mad Cowboy: Plain Truth from the Cattle Rancher Who Won't Eat Meat.* Lyman, H.F., with Merzer, G. Scribner. (2001).

9. *Empty Cages: Facing the Challenge of Animal Rights.* Regan, T. Rowman & Littlefield Publishers, Inc. (2004).

10. *Fast Food Nation: The Dark Side of the All-American Meal.* Schlosser, E. Perennial. (2002).

11. "What Meat Means." *New York Times.* Section 4, February 6, 2005.

12. *Vegan: The New Ethics of Eating, Revised Edition.* Marcus, E. McBooks Press. (2000).

13. *Beyond Beef: The Rise and Fall of the Cattle Culture.* Rifkin, J. Plume Books. (1993).

14. "What's the stench? A pile of cow manure 2,000-ton mountain of dung burns for 3 months in Nebraska town." The Associated Press. January 28, 2005.

15. *Hungry For Trade : How the Poor Pay for Free Trade.* Madeley, J. Zed Books. (2001).

16. *The Vegan Diet As Chronic Disease Prevention: Evidence Supporting the New Four Food Groups.* Saunders, K. Lantern Books. (2003).

17. *Carbophobia: The Scary Truth About America's Low-carb Craze.* Greger, M., M.D.. Lantern Books. (2005).

18. *The China Study : The Most Comprehensive Study of Nutrition Ever Conducted and the Startling Implications for Diet, Weight Loss and Long-Term Health.* Campbell, T.C., Campbell, T.M. Benbella Books. (2005).

19. *Food for Life : How the New Four Food Groups Can Save Your Life.* Barnard, N. Three Rivers Press. (1994).

20. *Becoming Vegan: The Complete Guide to Adopting a Healthy Plant-Based Diet.* Davis, B, Melina, V. Book Publishing Company (TN). (2000).

21. *Eat Right, Live Longer : Using the Natural Power of Foods to Age Proof Your Body.* Barnard, N., M.D. Harmony. (1995).

chapter three:
hell is
other people

We once heard someone say that "Everybody has an uncle Bill."
Okay, maybe you don't really have an uncle named "Bill," but
we're willing to bet there's someone in your life who's just like
Bob's Uncle Bill, or "UB" as we call him. UB is the uncle who lives for
a good fart joke, subscribes to *Penthouse* and *Playboy*, hates political cor-
rectness of all stripes, and has little regard for anything that seems different, un-American, or exotic. Though he's been diagnosed with high
cholesterol, high blood pressure, and other problems, he continues to
smoke, eats whatever the hell he wants, and laughs at anyone—including his doctors—who says pork rinds, hamburgers, and cigarettes are
bad for you. In the end, UB would likely drink his own urine before he
even thought of touching soymilk.

The question is, how do you deal with the UB in your life when
he starts hassling you for being a vegan? In our case, the hassle came
after last year's Christmas dinner at the home of Bob's parents. Having negotiated a vegan Christmas dinner without major arguments, we
thought we'd cleared the hurdles. After stuffing ourselves on good vegan
food, we reclined in our chairs and rested on our laurels. "Damn," we
thought to ourselves, "we're good!" We'd worked our way through another holiday without an argument over food and "how damn difficult

we are to please" (actual words of Bob's mom), and were completely self-assured of our vegan diplomatic prowess. We'd not only made our wishes known, but we'd done so without an argument, protestations, or other problems that often plague vegans around the very meat-centered holidays we do so love in America.[1]

Sitting back in our chairs enjoying our relative holiday success with a warm mug of coffee with soymilk, UB sidled up to the table, made a face, and picked up the soymilk carton.

Awww shit, here it comes...

UB, the great Archie Bunker of Philadelphia, was now eyeing the soymilk. As the very idea of soymilk registered in his brain, you could see his expression change from a smirk to utter disgust. Putting the carton down like it was a rat with bubonic plague, UB said "I'd rather enjoy what I eat and die young than drink this shit. All this healthy crap out there...who the hell wants it? You don't really like this shit, do you?"

At this point, the one thing you have to realize is that Bob isn't the kind of guy to run from an argument. In fact, some sick little part of him enjoys annoying people for sport, which is why many people have told him over the years that he'd make a great lawyer. Having had the "enemy" engage, Bob seemed ready to pounce. Actually, if Jenna was right, Bob was looking forward to pouncing.

"Yeah, we drink it. You should try it, it is pretty good," Bob replied in a friendly tone. Truth be told, Bob surprised even himself with this move. In the past, whenever anyone had challenged his vegetarian ways, he'd hunker down for an extended fight on the grounds of health, the environment, and animal rights. Bob is a real bastard if you cross him, and he never lets up. But somehow, on this day, Bob had matured beyond the skate-punk "fuck off" ethos, at least temporarily. And it worked.

---

1. Why is it that on every holiday we have to celebrate by slaughtering untold millions of animals to feed ourselves?

"Yeah, well, I'll never try that stuff," UB said, putting down the carton. Then he walked away.

That's right. He walked away. No more jokes. No more teasing. No more stupid cuts on vegetarians—nothing. By not getting upset over a stupid crack about soymilk, Bob denied UB the chance to get a rise out of us, something which he'd enjoy immensely. Since he tried and got nowhere with us, the game lost its appeal, and he immediately sensed there'd be no point in pushing it much further, particularly with so many offensive ethnic jokes waiting in the wings.

Naturally, not all confrontations go like this. Many of us get into heated arguments with people, and sometimes people just plain don't let up with their anti-vegan stupidity. Sometimes, we're pissed off, or worn down, or just plain tired of being called "plant killers." Whatever the case, there are times that we all feel like screaming at ignorant omnivores. Often, there's not much point in it, and in this chapter, we're going to explain why. We'll also explain the times we do feel it is worth griping, and we'll do a bit of griping ourselves along the way.

As a new vegan or someone who's thinking about becoming vegan, you might be wondering how to deal with family, friends, and co-workers. In this chapter, we're going to talk about how to get along with people while still being true to your ethics and choices. Along the way, we'll give you concrete advice about how to handle certain situations, and provide more philosophical advice about the appropriateness of being a member of the "vegan police." We'll also give you advice about how to get along with people you thought might never give you any heat at all: ovo-lacto vegetarians.

Repression

Before we get into how to deal with omnivores or carnivores or high-protein diet converts or whatever you want to call people who love meat, we'd like to take a quick foray into the mind of your average meat-eater. We're not aiming to be offensive, but we do want to give you a sense of what we see as the likely mental machinery that's necessary to eat meat without thinking too much about where it comes from. We do this not to be dismissive towards meat-eaters (many of whom can be wonderfully supportive of your veganism), but to give you a sense of where some of them might be coming from. Hopefully, this will help you react to them more effectively. Surely, every meat-eater is different, and we don't mean to suggest that this is a comprehensive way of understanding every single one, but we think this basic mental machinery is the basis of much of the guilt-free meat-eating that we see today, so bear with us for a bit, even if you think we might be full of shit. And hey—you probably already bought the book, so what do you have to lose?

In day-to-day situations, it has become abundantly clear to us that most people are simply not ready to hear the truth about their food just yet—particularly while they're eating. They don't want to know that veal calves are tortured and left in the dark from almost their first day on the face of the earth, or that layer hens are stacked seven to a tiny cage for their entire lives. As consumers, we possess an impressive repressive machinery that has its roots in the way that we're raised in capitalist, Western culture. Meat-eaters or not, we generally don't think much about where anything we consume comes from. Those who produce what we consume generally benefit greatly from this willful ignorance. Ultimately, this means that those who are directly involved in production can generally toil away in horrid conditions (and the more horrid the conditions, the lower the price) to make cheap shit that we can buy at WalMart. Our cheap sneakers come at the cost of exploiting labor somewhere down the line. Similarly, our cheap meat, eggs, and dairy come not only from exploiting animals, but also exploiting and dehumanizing the people that are involved in the production of these commodities. Just as we "innocently" presume that the person who made our cheap sneakers is being paid fairly for their work, we often "innocently" presume that animal agriculture operates with the welfare of animals and workers in mind. From the previous chapter, we know it doesn't. In both cases, there are examples where there's more rather than less justice for the oppressed and exploited, but these examples are few and far between.

More often than not, horrid, barbaric things are done to make a few extra dollars, and unfortunately, there's no shortage of people ready to exploit animals—human and non-human—for a few pennies more profit. Sadly, most of us are ready to buy what they produce. And of course, there's a related question of whether ignorance truly is bliss, or even a valid excuse.

The point here is that in capitalist cultures, we're acculturated to see only *things* and not to see the relationships that went into producing those things. This applies to our food as readily as it does to any other product. As a vegan, you complicate this relationship by reminding people there's something wrong at the heart of the matter when it comes to animals. Having seen beyond the pale of the product, having peered into the other side of suffering, exploitation, and death, we know meat is dead, and every sip of milk and every bite of egg contains within it suffering beyond words. To us, these products look dead, and for many vegans they arouse disgust and even nausea.

The problem is that we possess information that everyone else doesn't have, or doesn't want to think about. Knowing what we know, we want to tell everyone, because many of us are convinced that if people knew the truth, a lot of them would severely limit their consumption of these products or abandon them altogether. To vegans, veal is nothing but pointless abuse and murder. To others, it is a delicacy, and this is where things get tough. When you breach this wall that separates meat eating from meat, you're breaching years and years of active repression of this knowledge. Most meat-eaters are completely decent human beings with real feelings and compassion, and because of this, many don't want to come to terms with where their meat comes from. They'd prefer to be "innocent" consumers, but intentionally or otherwise, we're there reminding them they're not. This is why we vegans have to be especially careful around meat-eaters[2].

When you approach meat-eaters about veganism, or you are approached about your veganism, think of meat-eaters as analogous to children who still believe in Santa. If they're made to think about their meat, most meat-eaters would like to think that there's no pain and suffering involved in their food and clothes. But in contemporary meat production, this is as much a fiction as Santa. Just like the kids who want Santa to be real, many meat-eaters will deny the truth when you tell them. Frequently, meat-eaters will go to real lengths to ensure you don't destroy the fragile but deep-seeded fiction for them. This will often include marginalizing, belittling, and berating you, as well as making you seem like, well, a vegan freak. If they can assure themselves there's something wrong with *you* then they can assure themselves there's something wrong with your facts and your arguments too, and conveniently ignore you.

~~~~~~

Keeping this basic background in mind, we want to lay down some important strategies you're going to see repeated throughout this chapter in various situations. Going against our desire to be forthright and not to sugar-coat horrible facts for people, most of these strategies are nevertheless effective and can be best in the long-term. Considering the aforementioned mental machinery, they generally preserve peace, and they help to keep you sane, which is important. To be clear, there's absolutely no question in our minds that the exploitation and oppression of animals in our society is worthy of every ounce—or, for our international readers, gram—of moral outrage that you can muster. The hard part is learning how to effectively channel that outrage and use its en-

---

2. Of course, there are meat-eaters who revel in the death involved in their food, but these folks are truly a minority, we think. Much of what you'll hear along these lines is bluster designed to make you feel marginalized.

ergy for improving things without getting up in people's faces, though there are times that's appropriate too.

Much of this advice comes from experience—sometimes hard-learned—but a healthy dose of it also comes from the excellent book by Carol Adams called *Living Among Meat-eaters*. We recommend you buy her book if you need more in-depth suggestions about how to deal with family, friends, and romantic relationships, as we'll provide only a few examples and suggestions we've found particularly relevant in this chapter. In her 300-plus page book, Adams goes much further than we can here, and she does so with an eloquence that makes us envious. In addition, Compassion Over Killing (http://www.cok.net) puts out an excellent guide on these issues, as does Vegan Outreach (http://www.veganoutreach.org). We highly recommend all of these resources.

Nevertheless, here's our basic gist: non-confrontational strategies work the best in situations where people are familiar to you. That means with friends, family, and people at work, you should avoid the hard-line animal rights rhetoric about murder, the flesh of animals, and so on. There's nothing inherently wrong with hard-line animal rights tactics or rhetoric, but these are tools that need to be used appropriately and in the right context. You don't use a screwdriver when a wrench is appropriate, and you shouldn't probably cop the hard-line shit when you're eating with friends and family. This advice comes not because we're afraid of confrontation or honesty—and we'll explore why you need to be honest and upfront on some things below—but because we've seen non-confrontational strategies work the best for both the vegan in question and for the overall portrait of veganism. Our goal is to make veganism as widespread and easily adoptable as possible, and these methods seem to help to that end. Think of it like this: you might lose small battles along the way, but your aim is to win the war.

Before we get into the advice, we'd like to make a quick note: because we use these pieces of advice in each section, it may seem like we're repeating ourselves. In some sense, we are, but the advice fits several situations. In addition, not everyone reads books front to back;

people jump around, skim, and read sections as they have time, so we thought it important to include it at the risk of repetition, particularly for a chapter like this. Enough of the disclaimers. Let's get to the advice. Here, in no particular order, are our words of advice for dealing with family, friends, and those close to you personally.

• **Don't fight or talk about veganism in depth while you're eating.** As we talked about above, dinner isn't the time to be literal about the death involved in someone's veal scallopini. This turns people off, makes them even more defensive about their choices, and gets people angry at YOU. Talking in brief and vague terms over dinner is best. Don't give up altogether; just put off the conversation for a more appropriate time. Something like, "I'd be glad to talk about it, but it would probably be better to do it after we eat," is usually effective.

• **Don't be preachy to the meat-eaters in your life.** If you adopt the moral high ground when you talk to meat-eaters, they'll quickly grow tired of you and shut you out. No one likes to be condescended to, preached at, or picked on. It creates anger, it divides you and the person in question, and it puts people on the defensive. It could also make them hostile towards veganism more generally. In short, don't be a crass, annoying pain in the ass.

• **At least initially, let people come to you about veganism.** Sometimes people have a genuine curiosity and would like to know more about what it is like to be a vegan, or they have a hard time understanding what being a vegan means. If people come to you with questions about veganism, answer them honestly. This doesn't mean that you can't be proactive about having a vegan potluck, organizing a vegan action group, or showing films about vegan issues. It just means that you shouldn't be preachy.

• **Be secure in your veganism.** One of the best advertisements for veganism is happy vegans. Don't complain about what you don't have or how little there is to eat. Show people that vegans can be happy and content with food. Most meat-eaters and many vegetarians view veganism as deprivation. There's nothing better to cement this misconception in their mind than your illustrating it to them by whining about how little you have to eat, or how much you're depriving yourself "for the animals."

• **Food wins people over.** Cook vegan meals for the people in your life and show them that vegan food is delicious. Remind people through food that we vegans eat more than sticks, twigs, apples, and random yard scrapings. Don't even mention that the food is vegan—just invite people over for dinner and feed them well. Alternately, if you have a group of friends who might be interested in trying it out, organize a vegan potluck (after you've defined exactly what veganism is for them), or take them to a fabulous vegan restaurant.

• **Try not to get upset when taunted.** Some people pick on vegetarians and vegans for sport. By now, we're all familiar with the taunts. We're plant-haters, broccoli killers, sentimental animal lovers, etc., etc., etc. Surely there isn't a vegan alive who hasn't had a meat-eater stab a piece of meat with their fork, jam the meat into their mouth, and make sounds of utter pleasure as they eat dead flesh. (The pathetic part about this is that every stupid ass that does it thinks they're the first person to ever do it.) At this point, remember there is a feedback loop: the more you respond, the more power you give the person doing the taunting, and the more they're likely to continue. There are some really sick shits out there who, because they couldn't find any elderly people to push into traffic, get their jollies from this kind of annoying behavior. If you react, you're giving them their fix. We know this can be a real challenge. For many of us, letting this kind of idiotic behavior go is difficult, but we guarantee you it is better for your mental health!

• **Don't expect anyone to take care of you.** We're forever grateful to Carol Adams for this insight that seems basic, but is actually quite important. For instance, if you're going to someone's house for a big group dinner, you shouldn't expect to be catered to. Feed yourself ahead of time if you think there won't be much for you at the dinner, and offer to bring a dish of your own to share, so you have at least one thing to eat.

• **Meek vegans suffer.** You can't expect people to take care of you, but you should make your dietary needs known, and be abundantly clear about it. Don't just tell people you're vegan: tell them you don't eat any animal products including fish, eggs, milk, honey, and cheese (surprisingly, many people don't think of cheese as an animal product). You need to be completely up front about veganism when food is involved, or else you're likely to suffer. You cannot be afraid to approach people about it. While it can be uncomfortable, and for the really shy out there, downright torturous, you have to make your needs known or you will suffer, and not even we will feel bad for you.

• **No brute force.** The difficult lesson we've learned over time is that brute-force tactics often backfire when it comes to family and friends. Lecturing your Aunt Edna about suffering on egg farms over an omelette is generally a complete clusterfuck in the works. It creates animosity by making your omelette-loving Auntie feel judged, and then she's just going to tune you out, get completely angry, or have her feelings hurt. There are times that harder-line tactics are appropriate, but these times are limited, and if you want to remain on good terms with people in your life, it is best to limit your use of these tactics with them.

Using the principles that we've outlined here, below we discuss some of the scenarios and problems you might face when it comes to you, veganism, and your family. We follow with sections on dealing with friends and co-workers.

Family (or, "Am I really related to these people?")

When Jenna was an emotionally frail teenager on the cusp of puberty, her grandmother used to like to tell her that her butt was big.

"My god, look at that butt. Don't you think it is getting big?" she'd ask, waving her hand in the air like she was fanning away a horrible smell.[3]

Though Grammy never meant to be mean, this is about the most emotionally explosive thing you can say to a girl who's just starting to

---

3. Obviously, Grammy had never listened to Sir Mix-A-Lot.

become conscious of her figure and her sexuality.

There are two points to this anecdote worth noting. First, because family is so close to you, they often feel they can tell you whatever is on their mind, even if it comes at the cost of insulting you. This is particularly true if the family member doing the telling is a parent or someone older (and being an adult doesn't mean you automatically escape this, either). Second, much like Jenna being particularly sensitive about criticism around puberty, new vegans undergo a big transition themselves, so they're also particularly sensitive. To some extent, this is true whether you're a meek and unassuming vegan or whether you enjoy confrontation and arguments. As you're just getting used to being a vegan, you may not even be comfortable enough to talk about your reasons for your change. Maybe you know the reasons yourself, but you're not quite ready to defend them vigorously. Or perhaps you just weren't expecting you'd get quite so much static about it.

Family can be the toughest thing about going vegan, and many vegans hesitate to announce their veganism to their family. Reactions range from support and outright acceptance, to neutral ambivalence, to more potentially difficult situations that include threats ("eat this or else..."), teasing ("mmmm....juicy steak"), and lengthy complaints and arguments ("you don't love my food so you don't love me"). Sadly, there's no single way to deal with these problems. Part of the issue at hand is that every family is different, and there is no such thing as a "normal" family. You have to work in a way that's going to be the most effective in your situation. Some of this may require rethinking ways you've dealt with family problems in the past, particularly if you've not had much luck resolving them, or you're prone to yelling matches. Your best bet in almost any case is to be firm but polite about your choices. You definitely should not lecture others on their choices, even if you find them completely horrifying. For a while, until everyone gets used to the idea, it can be difficult. But you can smooth things over by offering to cook for your family on occasion (some people are honestly floored by how good vegan food can be), offering to prepare your own food if necessary, and, if you can, buying your own groceries.

Whatever you do, you should not back down from your choice to be a vegan. Don't be intimidated and cowed into doing something you disagree with. You have to live for yourself, and you have to live with your choices. This means you should not take mini-vacations from veganism to make people happy or avoid conflict. All this does is delay the problem, showing your family you're not really serious about what you're doing. On top of all of this, if they used coercive methods to get you to drop your veganism—however briefly—it shows them coercion works. Remember: meek vegans suffer.

One place where all of this can be particularly intense can be around holidays, but the same basic rules apply. If you can stand to be around meat enough to be at a table with meat-eaters, your best bet is to bring your own food, particularly if whomever is cooking isn't making something vegan for you. If being around turkey carcasses or ham (or whatever) really bothers you, you'll have to draw that line and stick to it for your own sanity. Again, you must decide what your boundaries are; then resolve to stick to them firmly but politely.

However, remember that being assertive doesn't mean you should rage against your family, call them animal killers, or splash fake blood on them when they eat meat. You may have to be somewhat less confrontational than you'd like, but this is the price you may have to pay if you want to maintain good relationships with your kin. As we've said earlier, there's no better advertisement for your certainty about veganism than your being secure in your choice and communicating that to others.

You should consider how food creates emotional attachments we wouldn't necessarily expect, and how food is also used to define roles. Bob's mom, for example, loves to cook for everyone. She loves having tons of people in the house, and she enjoys feeding them until they're on the verge of bursting. Knowing this, people do indeed come from all around the neighborhood to eat, because Bob's mom always has plenty around, and if she doesn't, she'll actually run out and get you something. This creates a welcoming environment and you can get fed incredibly well.

The problem is that by becoming vegan, Bob complicated this role for his mother. In his veganism, he made it more difficult for her to find fulfillment by preparing tons upon tons of food for him. What once was an enjoyable thing for her became an annoying challenge. "What can I make ya, hon?" became "Jesus Christ, you are so goddamn impossible to please!"

In all honesty, Bob's mom has been pretty supportive of our decision to be vegan, but initially it threw her off when it came to her expertise as a cook and as a provider, and because Bob's relationship with food changed, Bob's relationship with his mom was also changing in subtle ways. After a few months, Bob's mom did buy a few vegan cookbooks, and now she's trying some new recipes (which is good news for us!). Still, it took some time to get to this point, and you shouldn't be surprised if someone in your life sees your refusal of certain foods as an affront to their cooking or them personally. Remember that you might be challenging a long-standing role and that any change takes time and patience if it is to be meaningful, particularly in parent-child relationships, regardless of age. It is best if you politely stand firm and explain your choices. Also, don't let emotional games from family members get in the way of your ethical decision. It is vital that you remain rational and that you not turn this situation into a screaming match or a battle of wills. Explain your reasons, let them know what you do and don't eat, and offer to cook your own food or to cook for the family every so often. Standing strong and showing them that you're serious about what you're doing is the best option. Some families will be incredibly supportive and some won't be, and how you negotiate this has to work within your family dynamics as appropriate. But don't forget the importance of your choice and why you've made it.

Another way that family tends to react to your veganism is by assuming it is just a "phase" that you're going through. There are two ways to read this reaction:

A) The Generous Reading

Perhaps readers of our generation went through a "phase" where they liked acid-washed jeans and Orchestral Manoeuvres in the Dark, or maybe they went through a "phase" where they wore parachute pants, beat-boxed, and saved their allowance for a square of linoleum for break dancing[4]. Or, maybe they went through a skate-punk phase that they never quite grew out of[5]. Whatever the case, these are legitimate fads. Like any other person, you probably got sucked into a few of them. But if you're vegan and vegan for the "right" reasons—as we discussed in Chapter 1—you're likely not into veganism as a fad, but as a deeper expression of your ethical choices. This is why there's simply no comparison between acid-washed jeans and veganism. However, that doesn't mean this is how your family will see it. To them, your newfound veganism is likely as capricious as your love of those god-awful hideous parachute pants. They didn't get why you wanted a square of linoleum for break dancing, and they probably don't get why you'd give up what they see as tasty and delicious animal products. So when you tell them you're a vegan or that you're going vegan, they probably read you through the lens of their own experience with you and your previous forays into territory they didn't necessarily "get."

B) The Ungenerous Reading

Your family assumes you're essentially incapable of making any long-standing decisions on your own, they view you as an immature child, and expect that your life is governed by fickle, ill-informed whims. Having made such silly choices from your heart and not with your logic, they expect that you'll eventually come around, see the light, and go back to your meat-eating, egg-sucking, milk-loving ways.

The problem, of course, is that A and B aren't mutually exclusive, but far be it from us to tell you which one is more common.

---

4. For the record, neither of us went through either of these phases. Honest. Do you think we'd ever admit to them so publicly if we did?

5. However, this phase Bob owns up to.

Though you might think we're aiming this at teenagers, this talk of "phases" can apply even to people who have grown up, gotten PhDs, and done other very adult things (hmmm...doesn't *that* sound dirty!). Jenna, who has indeed grown up, gotten her PhD, and taken on a full-time job, still regularly gets asked by her parents if she's "still a vegan." Though Jenna's parents are pretty cool about her veganism, their understanding seems to operate on the principle that her veganism is temporary. Part of this probably has to do with reading Jenna's awesome, rad, and completely gnarly 80s phase as a fad, but another part of this has to do with them seeing veganism as nothing but deprivation. To them and many omnivores, veganism looks like the worst kind of diet. For a lot of omnivores, life without animal products just seems not worth living, as pathetic as that seems to us on the flip side. Coming from this angle, they'll view veganism as some kind of diet with near-religious strictures and wonder how anyone could keep at it for so very long. The best way to deal with this is to stick to your beliefs.

One final point before we close this section on family. Challenges to your veganism from family can come as "concerns about your health." You'll hear the familiar litany of perceived problems: "how will you get your calcium/protein/iron?" "Will you die if you don't eat meat?" "Can you just live on vegetables alone?" "Aren't humans meant to eat meat?"[6]

To answer these questions, we highly recommend the book *Becoming Vegan: The Complete Guide to Adopting a Healthy Plant-Based Diet* by Brenda Davis and Vesanto Melina. The authors are experts on vegan nutrition and their book includes a variety of chapters that deal with questions of vegan nutrition. Even if you don't get hassled by your family about veganism and nutrition, this is a good one to pick up because it can give you a sense of how to eat well as a vegan.

---

6. A friend of ours actually solved this very problem by offering to see a nutritionist, but only if the whole family saw one. It worked well for him because the nutritionist explained that a balanced vegan diet was healthy, and that was the end of it.

With some work, most families can be pretty flexible and come to see your choices as valid. In time, they'll probably even respect you for your commitment. It might take work, persistence, patience, and a saintly humility on your part, but eventually, they're likely to come around. After all, they're your family, and you're stuck with them and they're stuck with you, so you should try to make it work.

Friends

Love 'em or hate 'em, they're the people that you spend your free time with, and you have to deal with them. At some point, you're bound to end up in a situation that involves eating, and you're going to have to talk about your veganism. If you're lucky, you have cool friends who are big-hearted, love you without question, and take your veganism into consideration when choosing a restaurant or preparing a meal.

If you're unlucky, your friends just suck. By "just suck" we mean that they think you're being insane. They may tease you, sabotage your veganism, and give you a hard time about being too difficult. Or perhaps they just look at you funny. Regardless, you have to be ready for the fact that your veganism can change the way that at least some of your friends and their families relate to you. You may be seen as unworkable and inconsiderate for asking that you go to a restaurant with vegetarian options, or even for politely turning down meat. Like others, your friends may assume that you're looking for attention, going too far with this "vegetarian thing" or just "going through a phase," or all of the above. Point is, you can't expect the reactions of your friends to be all that different than the reactions of the rest of the world on this matter, even if your friends are among the most accepting people in other areas[7].

---

7. As we mentioned in Chapter 2, it is worth noting that "liberals" or "leftists" can be generally accepting of vegans, but often, they'll give you lip about animal rights because they think that you're not "putting people first." This is complete bunk, because often these people aren't even putting people first themselves, and on top of it all, there's nothing that says that one cannot simultaneously fight against the exploitation of both human and non-human animals. We say this as committed leftists. So there.

Our advice is simple on this account. You should always be up front with your friends about your veganism. We'll say it yet again: **meek vegans suffer!** If friends are throwing a dinner party, it is best if you get in touch with them ahead of time to tell them you're vegan. You should explain exactly what this means in clear terms (e.g., "I don't eat meat, eggs, dairy, or fish."). It isn't that we think your friends are dumb, but you can't assume that everyone knows what veganism is. If you make this assumption, you might end up sitting in front of a dish covered in cheese. Offer to bring something with you, because then at least you have one thing to eat if all else fails[8]. And if you think there won't be much for you to eat, just have a bite ahead of time so that you aren't starving.

When you offer to bring your own food, you remove the burden for the host if she was planning on cooking stuffed buffalo head or whatever the latest gourmet torture-filled dish of the week is. You're also playing a subtle game here: if you bring a vegan dish to share and it really rocks, then you can show others than veganism isn't just about eating yard scrapings, which is what many people suspect and fear. If you use recipes from good cookbooks, you can show them that vegan food can be creative, delicious, and artful despite their initial misgivings. If you are taking a dish, it is best to take something that looks and tastes good, unless you really just want to eat the whole thing yourself (which is okay too).

If you're lucky enough to have friends like ours, they'll likely make something special for you or change the whole menu to make you feel more welcomed. Or maybe you have so many vegetarian and vegan friends that at your next dinner party you'll put the meat-eater in the minority position for a change. This can be great fun, because then you can pepper them with dumb questions. Many of our friends are vegetarians or vegans, but we do have meat-eating friends as well. When we cook for our meat-eating friends, they often seem surprised by how good

---

8. Though this can backfire: if what you bring is really good, everyone might eat it, and you'll be stuck with next to nothing. You might keep a back-up reserve in the car, if possible, or eat ahead of time.

the food is[9], again because they imagine that what we do is all about sacrifice, which it isn't. It can be fun to pleasantly surprise people.

On the other hand, maybe your friends aren't so receptive. Maybe they're the kind that hit you with the million hypothetical situations ("would you eat meat if..."), chew steak loudly in your face, yell at you, hide meat or dairy in your food, or give you a really hard time about being too difficult. In this case, our advice is again simple: tell them this is your choice, and you expect them to respect it. Give them some time to come around, but don't tolerate too much bullshit, particularly if they're hiding non-vegan things in your food. Be firm but polite, and don't let the teasing get to you. You should stand up for yourself, but don't get sucked into stupid arguments, especially while you're eating.

Also, you may or may not want to flip the tables on people who give you shit. For example, Bob was once having lunch with a student of his named Phyllis when he ordered the soy riblet sandwich. Knowing Bob was a vegan, Phyllis looked at the sandwich with disgust, saying, "Eww, Bob, how can you eat that? It looks like something I'd feed my dog." Bob looked back at her egg and cheese sandwich with the same disgust and said "Eww, Phyllis, how can you eat cow puss and all of those chicken reproductive excretions?" Having completely grossed Phyllis out, Bob turned her off of her sandwich completely. The point of this story isn't to say that you should do this often. Though it can be wildly fun to throw back a little jibe here and there when you're annoyed with someone, turning the tables like this can be dangerous, and we don't often recommend it. Every so often, though, you may just need to do a little vegan self-defense (ve-gan-do) for your own health and sanity. We've found that repeated annoyances by meat-eaters are often thwarted by discussions of *E. coli* or mad cow disease.

If you've been patient, polite, and non-harassing, and your friends *still* give you shit about being a vegan, you might need to find new friends. Maybe this sounds harsh, but if you're into veganism for the long haul and you're serious about your ethics, you need to have friends

---

9. This is cool at first, but when you think about it, it can be a bit insulting later, no?

who support your decision without giving you crap. The occasional bust or joke isn't anything to "dump" friends over, but if you're constantly being bombarded with stupid comments and the like, you need to make a stand, tell your friends how you feel, and tell them they need to stop. If they don't take you seriously, there's likely something wrong with your relationship, and apart from psychological issues that we can't really diagnose, there's no reason to stay in a relationship—friendly or otherwise—that is abusive. Veganism is a big part of any vegan's life, and those close to you should respect it.

Whether you're in a bad situation with your friends or not, you can likely find support and more vegan company in local vegetarian or vegan societies. If you live in a city in the US or Canada, you can also meet vegan folks through dinners and other events organized via http://vegan.meetup.com. Though we've never been to a meet-up, we hear that they're pretty cool. There are meet-ups in cities all across the US and Canada. For those of you who might be suspicious, we should note that this isn't an online dating service; it is simply a way for vegans to meet other vegans and hang out. If you are interested in a dating service that caters specifically to vegans or vegetarians, you might have a look online. VegWeb (http://www.vegweb.com) currently runs an inexpensive service, and you can surely find others with the help of Google.

Romance aside, if you're in college or even just a college town, you can probably find other vegans pretty easily in a campus vegan or animal rights group, or through the local co-op (if it isn't loaded with wealthy, middle-aged ex-hippies who are too busy worrying about the international cause du jour to pay attention to something like veganism). Many campuses have vegan or vegetarian groups that hold get-togethers and potlucks. Some groups even sponsor local actions, leafletting, and protests. If your campus does not have an active vegan group, we'd encourage you to start one. All you need to do is come up with a name, spend a few bucks photocopying flyers (or get your friend at the copy center to do them for free) announcing a meeting time and place, and show up and see what people want to do. It really can be just that simple. Another thing that helps getting the group off the ground is setting up a free email list at Yahoo! or GoogleGroups to keep everyone informed of events and actions on campus and in the area.

In the case of the campus where we work, a few dedicated students were able to put together a Vegan Action Group in the course of a few weeks and gain permanent status for the club after a semester. Our local Vegan Action Group was able to get University funding to show films like *The Witness* and *Peaceable Kingdom,* and to host an evening where anyone could come and try vegan foods for free. The group grew quickly, even on our relatively conservative and apolitical campus, and as a consequence, members of the group were able to successfully lobby the school cafeterias for more vegan dishes.

If you do start a vegan group, it is important you don't close it off to anyone. Accept all people, omnivorous, vegan, and otherwise, and give them a chance to explore things without pressure. Answer their questions honestly, and let them come to veganism at their own speed. Of course, if a more dedicated subset of the group wishes to do more radical actions, stage protests, or push things further (however defined), that subset of the group is always free to do so, with or without the express blessing of the larger group. This is up to you and your group to decide. Sometimes, depending on the context, more radical action is appropriate and essential. Still, remember you are always a representative for veganism and/or animal rights activists, and whatever you do will be used to judge *all* vegans and/or animal rights activists. Though we think that radical action has a place, we would encourage you to think carefully about the repercussions of your actions, and work from there.

When it comes down to it, dealing with friends is pretty much like dealing with anyone else: you need to balance your forthrightness with some flexibility, and sometimes you have to take some shit you otherwise might not want to put up with. But when it does come down to it, most of your friends will likely come around to at least a passing acceptance of your veganism. Remember: it pays to be polite but firm, to stand up for yourself, and to avoid lecturing. With some luck and perseverance, you'll be able to get along just fine with your non-vegan friends.

We've dealt with friends and we've dealt with family, but this still leaves at least one other group of omnivores to talk about. Unless you're lucky enough to be independently wealthy, you also have to deal with those who slave along with you for 40-plus hours a week in the interests of "the man." In the next section, we provide advice on dealing with co-workers, bosses, and others at that dreaded place where we turn our time into money: work!

Does Somebody Have a Case of the Mondays?

You're at your company's annual BBQ and you're politely declining the charred meat on the grill. You're at the cafeteria desperately searching for something other than salad. You get invited to lunch with your co-workers and you try to suggest going for Chinese or Indian so you can eat something other than french fries. You're sitting in your office quietly eating the lunch you brought from home. In any case, just by trying to eke out an existence in the world of omnivores, you once again become the vegan freak.

During one of these vegan freak moments, Jenna was just trying to get through the end-of-the-semester department dinner without making too much of a scene. After all, they're the people you have to see every day and who have a say in your future employment, so you don't want to totally freak them out. In years past, the dinner was buffet-style, so there wasn't such a focus on the food at hand. This year, however, it was a sit down dinner—bad news. Luckily, Jenna thought ahead and asked the secretary to order her a vegan meal, because damn if she was going to pay $25 for a meal and not be able to eat any of it. But because it was a sit down dinner, Jenna's veganism suddenly became much more conspicuous. As everyone headed toward the dining room, Jenna heard "Hey, Jenna, your dinner is on its way!"

Because the kitchen nearly forgot about the vegan meal, it came later than everyone else's, drawing even more attention. When it arrived, the inevitable questions started. "So you're a vegan..." Just as this question came, another person asked what a vegan is. Jenna patiently explained that she doesn't eat any meat, dairy, or eggs. "So where do you get your protein? Your calcium? You're young now, but it's never too early to think about osteoporosis." Given this, Jenna wanted desperately to launch into a discussion of how vegan diets actually are *better* at preventing osteoporosis because they have plenty of calcium, and too much animal protein leaches calcium out of your bones, but she bit her tongue and gave the standard answer "it's no problem to get protein and calcium" and mumbled something about beans, tofu and leafy greens. "So are you vegan for political reasons or some other reason?" Jenna responded briefly, saying "for animal rights reasons primarily, and secondarily for health." Then for some reason the discussion turned to the South Beach diet and how yummy free-range meat is, although bison is apparently a little bland. One person even made the comment that "I guess happy animals taste better." Jenna again desperately wanted to shout "they'd be a lot fucking happier if you didn't eat them!" but since the focus was off her, she instead carried on a conversation about gardening and herbs with the person sitting next to her.

Although we are extremely proud to be vegans and would gladly have a discussion with anyone interested, work is another realm where you have to learn to pick your battles or you'll end up going crazy and ostracize yourself from others, rather than having the chance to show others how great being a vegan can be. As we've already stated, being confrontational can sometimes be a good thing, but you have to read the situation and figure out if it's worth it. Once you reveal yourself as a vegan at work, you are going to get a lot of different reactions. Some people are very accommodating, even overly so. Others will ask you the familiar stupid questions that will drive you nuts and try your patience every time. Some will tag you as a freak and make fun of you or even try to get you to eat meat, just like family and friends. A lot of what goes on depends on the kind of work you do and the setting in which you work. Hardly anyone would even notice that Jenna is a vegan in her department if it weren't for group dinners and get togethers. Other people have to deal with cafeterias, communal lunch areas, or going out to eat with clients or co-workers on a regular basis.

As with family and friends, with co-workers it's important to remember the guidelines outlined above. Discussions about veganism at work will most likely come up over food, so being confrontational may be detrimental to the image others have of vegans. Make your wishes known ahead of time if possible (again, meek vegans suffer!), and always be solid in and happy about your commitment to being vegan.

These general recommendations can play out in any number of ways in the workplace, depending on what type of environment you work in. The best advice we can give you is to bring your own food (like lunches and snacks) to work since you'll know it is vegan. If you're organized, you can make a large batch of rice, pasta, soup, sandwich filling, or salad-type dish on the weekend and take portions of it during the week. We know this sounds soccer-mom-like, but trust us—it is worth it, especially if you want to eat healthy and not be starving by dinner time every day, or if you want to avoid spending lots of money at a restaurant. Bring little containers of applesauce, pretzels, vegan jerky, fruit, carrots, hummus, or whatever else floats your boat for snacks so you don't always have to rely on the vending machine (remember, you can't read the ingredients before you buy!), cafeteria, or local restaurants or stores. All of this will probably save you money in the long run too, since it is cheaper than eating out. The authors of the cookbook *Garden of Vegan* suggest finding a funky lunchbox to bring your food in that has a thermos for soup, so you can be environmentally sound and cool at the same time. Hey, your mom might still have your Strawberry Shortcake or Masters of the Universe lunchbox laying around from when you were a kid.

Jenna found one unique plus to taking her own lunches every day—people starting asking questions and being interested in what she brought. As soon as she was done heating her lunch in the microwave, the secretary would say, "Oh, that smells good! What is it?" and even sometimes ask for the recipe. If people understand what it is that vegans actually do eat (see chapter 4 for more on this), they can start to grasp that we're not all malnourished freaks.

If you have to eat in a cafeteria, you might still be able to bring your own lunch and sit with your co-workers. If your cafeteria is vegan friendly, you're lucky. If not, you can ask to speak with the staff who run the cafeteria and request that they provide a vegan option every day. You'd be surprised—people might be more accommodating than you'd expect. Or, they'll tell you politely to go to hell and eat the damn salad. Make sure they understand the difference between being vegan and vegetarian, so you don't end up with a cheese-laden dish. (Again, mention milk, butter, mayonnaise, cheese, cream, honey, etc. since people tend to forget that products other than the obvious have dairy and/or eggs.) If you expect that they won't be accommodating, phrase it as if you "can't have" something, rather than "won't eat" something. If people think you have an allergy, fine. It's sad that people will be more tolerant of an unintentional choice rather than a conscious dietary choice, but that's the way it is. In some situations it might be necessary to take this approach so you're assured a nice meal or that the staff won't piss in your food.

Going out to eat with co-workers or clients provides another challenge, which is discussed in detail in chapter 4. One possibility that we mentioned above is that you try to get everyone to go to a Chinese, Indian, or other type of restaurant that you know will likely have at least one vegan entree, rather than going to a steakhouse, having to smell all that dead flesh, and eating nothing but a baked potato without butter. Bob has used this strategy with success to go to a Chinese buffet rather than a deli with his colleagues. If you're somewhere where you don't have much to choose from, then eat what you can and grab something afterwards. Answer any questions that come up politely and just say "no thank you" if someone offers you something you don't want to eat. Don't get into a fight during the meal. And last but not least, don't look miserable. This might be hard to do if you have irritating co-workers, but it's worth it to try. Don't make it look like you have to suffer to be a vegan, even though you know it's annoying as all hell to be in a restaurant that doesn't cater to vegans.

These suggestions also apply to special dinners or BBQs at someone's house. Like when you deal with your friends, you can ask politely beforehand if there will be anything you can eat, and don't force the person to make you something special (they'll likely be clueless as to what to offer you anyway). Offer to bring your own dish, or just show up with your own veggie burgers if it's a BBQ. The last resort is that you eat before you go and just enjoy the company you're with rather than sharing their meal.

As we saw with family, friends, and co-workers, being vegan around non-vegans can be a test of your diplomatic prowess, not to mention your patience. But trust us, from experience we have found that being non-confrontational with people you have to deal with on a regular basis can actually open their eyes—even if just a little—to veganism. And if you think it's all bad, we need to mention that we have had some wonderfully accommodating friends and family that have provided us with great vegan meals, even though we insisted that we could bring something on our own. As time goes on, people may become more receptive and even go out and buy some vegetarian cookbooks, as our parents did.

Before we finish our chapter on dealing with others, we need to discuss some other people that you may encounter who might challenge your veganism: ovo-lacto vegetarians and ex-veg*ns[10].

---

10. Veg*n is often used to designate vegetarians and vegans together (the '*' is a wild-card character on most computer systems).

Dealing with Vegetarians

One of the last places where you'd expect any hostility about your veganism is from ovo-lacto vegetarians, pesectarians, or others who seem (at least on the surface) to hold kindly views towards vegetarianism in general. In our experience, the vast majority of ovo-lacto vegetarians are completely cool about veganism, but there are a minority of ovo-lacto vegetarians who will enjoy harassing you or will view you with suspicion and doubt. They'll scan you for leather (even though they may be wearing it), quiz you on the extent of your veganism, and look for cracks in the foundation of your veganism. They may call you a radical, or dismiss you for going "too far" with your vegetarianism. After all, in their minds, why would you be a vegan when milk and eggs don't directly kill animals (and they taste 'oh-so-good')?

In some ways, this kind of reaction isn't all that much different than what hostile meat-eaters sometimes do to attack us, and that's not a co-incidence. In both cases, the ultimate goal is to be able to dismiss us and our choices through a constant dissection. If they can break us down in even one place and show us not to be the pinnacle of compassionate perfection that they expect, then they can dismiss us, at least in their own heads. Somehow, if they can trip us up, they can call us hypocrites, and return to eating their Eggs Benedict.

Another part of what's going on here is a feeling that we're being judgmental. Granted, some vegetarians do have run-ins with judgmental vegans who annoyed the hell out of them, but we know enough vegans to confidently say that preachy vegans are a tiny minority in the world of vegan freakdom. Even if you aren't being preachy, you can still be perceived as someone who thinks that they're better than everyone else, only because you're doing something different than vegetarians. In essence, your choice to avoid what they're eating is perceived as judging *them*. When vegetarians meet you and learn that you're vegan, they're forced to remember why it is that they're vegetarian, and they have to ultimately confront why they're not vegan too. In that instant, your very presence has likely forced them into some tough thinking. All at once, they've got to come to terms with why they're not vegan, decide if it is something that they're interested in or not, and then also decide how to react to you. If they're really into their cheese/milk/eggs/etc., then the initial reaction may be something like "wow, I'm a vegetarian, but I could never be a vegan. I just don't think I could ever live without my cheese/milk/eggs/etc." This is an understandable reaction, particularly if the person doesn't know many vegans or understand the ethics behind veganism.

Other ovo-lacto vegetarians may want to paint you as the freak (yet again). As we mentioned above, if they can conveniently put you into a category of "radical" or "freak" in their brains, then they can adequately dismiss you, and subsequently, dismiss your choices too. Ovo-lacto vegetarians have actually asked us, "Don't you think you're taking this just a bit too far?" This is their way of sticking you into a little box that they can deal with and conveniently ignore. Against our expectations, this kind of reaction is more intense in 'mixed' company of omnivores and vegetarians, when the vegetarian doesn't want to be seen as marginal, radical, and far-out as you. It is the way the vegetarian communicates to the rest of the group "Hey, I'm okay, I'm not nearly as weird as the vegan!"

So, how does one respond to these kinds of problems? There's a lot to be said for standing up from the table, giving everyone the finger, and flipping the table over as you run out of the room calling everyone "murderers" and proclaiming the need for animal liberation.

Or perhaps not.

Seriously, the best way we've found to deal with this is to just let it go. That goes against our ethos most of the time, which is generally to say what's on our minds regardless of the consequences, but in this case, it won't help (just like we describe above in our encounters with family, friends, and co-workers). One of the best responses we've found is a simple, "This is my choice and it might not be right for you, but I feel better this way. If you're curious, I'd be happy to talk to you about it." Surprisingly, something that simple can be incredibly effective and even disarming.

It bears mention here that if you're already a vegan, you should be kind to vegetarians regardless of what you think of their choices. We're not saying you should collapse if confronted on the question of animal cruelty and how it relates to eggs and milk, but we are saying you should maybe think twice before getting frustrated. One characteristic common to all vegans is that we're passionate about what we're doing. We're the "converted," in a sense. We take our choice to be the sensible one, and some of us get frustrated when we see others not doing what we know is right. We've seen a great shirt on the "Internets" that has the word "Vegetarian" with the "etari" cut out (resulting in the word "vegan") and the slogan underneath it says something like "Cut out the crap. Go Vegan." We think this sums up how many vegans feel, but we can't forget that *the vast majority of vegans were vegetarians first.* If we do forget and get pissed at vegetarians for not coming around quickly enough, we run the risk of being judgmental idiots who scare people off of the good thing that veganism is.

In our case, we've found ourselves annoyed beyond words with vegetarians who've sat in a room with us after a lecture decrying the horrors of the dairy industry that they continue to support through their consumption of—get this—MILK PRODUCTS! Grr. We wanted to stand up, give them the middle finger, flip the table over... oh, wait, sorry...ummm, we actually wanted to stand up on our chairs and scream at them, "HOW CAN YOU KNOW THIS AND STILL DRINK MILK, YOU COMPLETE IDIOT?" but decided against it. (Can you tell that we like the idea of standing up on stuff to make a point?) Had we done this, we'd be nothing better than the unpleasant judgmental vegan, we'd be asking someone to make a choice on *our* terms rather than their own, and we'd probably be fucking up this person's possible movement towards veganism on their own terms (which is the only way to go, we think). We're not going to lie: we want everyone to be vegan, we're working towards that, and we do a lot towards helping people move in this direction in our activism. But yelling at people, calling them on their contradictions, and challenging them isn't always the best way to approach the issue. For one, it personalizes things in ways that aren't always helpful and makes people feel attacked and marginalized. For another, it makes you look like a complete bastard with nothing better to do and it lets people dismiss both you and veganism. Our friend Dan Peyser (who we mentioned in Chapter 1) says it best: "Remember, people are often led to become vegan by the example of others. Don't fuck it up by being an annoying twat about it."

Like mom used to say, patience is a virtue. Rather than getting angry at ovo-lacto vegetarians for "going halfway" or not being committed enough to animal liberation causes, continue to educate them about animal exploitation and oppression when it is appropriate. We let people come to us on their terms, and then from there, we work with them as their interest dictates. Again, it sometimes goes against our very real desire to scream sense into people, but we've found this to be more effective. This less confrontational strategy works because there are a number of thoughtful vegetarians who will never stop thinking about veganism after they've come to discover that it is possible, with you as an example. For others, they may never get beyond where they're at, but in this world of limited time and resources, your energies towards vegan activism are best spent on those who have the best chance of becoming vegan rather than badgering the hell out of someone who will likely never make the step. In either case, it can't hurt to cook for them if you're halfway decent at it.

Before we call it quits for this section, there's yet one more kind of vegetarian annoyance to deal with: the unrepentant ex-vegetarian or ex-vegan. We're not talking about folks who were once vegetarian and now want to return to vegetarianism; if nothing else, these people are usually your friends. No, we're talking about a different kind of creature, a different kind of beast born of weakened and misplaced commitment. We're talking about the loudmouthed ex-vegan.

Unfortunately, ex-vegans have a way of popping up at the most inopportune times, more often than not when you're being asked about your veganism by omnivores. Explaining what you do and don't eat and why, you might find yourself interrupted by the busybody ex-vegan who makes it her job to tell everyone why she's not vegan anymore. This usually goes along with a loud and long-winded explanation of why she thinks veganism is absurd and unworkable. This kind of vigilante ex-veganism is a direct blow to you because it makes *you* look absurd and unworkable. As the ex-vegan plies your omnivorous company with tales of why he "just can't give up burgers" or how he "must eat sashimi" (the yuppie scum), you come out looking like the freak (again!). They make you look like their former bad choice manifest in bodily form like some kind of ghost of veganism past. Plus, they make veganism seem like a fad diet, the granola and whole-grain version of Atkins®, or whatever the pop fad diet is this week on Oprah. On top of it all, they basically imply that veganism is just a silly phase.

When the ex-vegan speaks up ever so loudly, they give your omnivorous company the permission to think of you as marginal, weird, and out there. You're being painted as a freak, and on some levels that's frustrating as hell. Even though you might have "FTW[11]" tattooed on your forehead and you don't really care what anybody thinks, at this point, you've likely started to lose whatever kind of legitimacy you might have had in the eyes of your omnivorous comrades.

If you haven't witnessed the odd voyeurism of soul-searching ex-veganism, you can find a prime example of it in the May 23rd 2005 edition of the *Village Voice* online. In an article titled "Where's the Beef?" Sloane Crosley details her "roughage exposé" (oh, how witty), comparing vegans to transsexuals (as if veganism is anywhere near that hard) and charting her own forays into veganism and vegetarianism. Now, she writes, she can't "hack it as a vegetarian" because:

---

11. For those of you not down with old-skool punk rock, "Fuck The World" tattoos were popular among those, who, well, thought little of the rest of the world.

"New York is sushi city, and sushi is the one thing that I've constantly craved over the past decade (besides the secret craving of every vegetarian: bacon). My education about the moral and environmental impact of eating meat is thorough, but my response to all the statistics has developed a major fissure called 'sashimi.'"

Though Crosley claims to avoid all other meat, she's given in to sushi because she thinks that claims of fish suffering are overblown (despite convincing evidence to the contrary). She's even gone as far as to lie to other vegetarians about her fish-eating, claiming that she "developed an iron deficiency." At the end of the article, she writes that she "still considers [herself] a vegetarian, but after this little confession the tofu mafia will cast [her] out."

There are a handful of problems here that need to be dealt with, but more than anything, this strikes me as the kind of broadside that's meant to make vegetarians—and vegans more specifically—look like ruthless fools. By aligning herself with people who eat sushi and fearing reprisal from the "tofu mafia," she paints us vegans as radical weirdos, which is good for her: by disassociating herself from us and cursing what she sees as our dietary inflexibility, she builds a comfortable space for herself. If she decides we're being too strict, she can subsequently dismiss us, just as she's done here. When she does so in such a public fashion, it makes us look intolerant to people who don't really have much real-world experience with vegans.

Crosley's article also brings up another point worth discussing here: namely, that FISH IS NOT A VEGETABLE. Yes, though we realize that many of our readers will be stunned—absolutely stunned—to read this, we have come to this ground-breaking conclusion through hours upon hours of careful research here in the Vegan Freak HQ high-tech science lab[12] using 4th grade science textbooks. Upon consultation with these sources, we have indeed discovered that fish are in fact in the biological kingdom called "ANIMALIA." One needn't have studied Latin extensively to understand that "animalia" is quite close to the English

---

12. Of course, no animals were harmed in this research.

word "animal." Damn Catholicism and its Friday no-meat-but-fish-is-okay guidelines for being the root of all of this confusion!

Point is, why call yourself a vegetarian (which she still does) if you continue to eat animals? If she gets upset because we vegans and vegetarians get pissed at her for eating fish, it is because veg*ns don't eat animals. Why is that so hard to get?

Vegan? Vegetarian? Does it Matter?

Along these lines, there seems to be some debate in the circles that we run in about whether the definition of vegan/vegetarian matters or not. Take the following example that we saw come across a mailing list that we're on: A woman lives on a farm where she raises her own chickens and harvests their eggs. Though she doesn't eat the eggs or animal products of any kind, she does harvest the eggs for her family, and she also slaughters the chickens for her family.

Now, ask yourself: is this woman a vegan?

Technically speaking, if this woman doesn't eat/use/wear animal products of any kind, she's a vegan, right? Some people say yes, others say no. Though she doesn't technically consume any animal products herself, she does enable others to do so, and on top of it all, she slaughters animals. Most of the ethical vegans argued that this woman may be *technically* vegan, but that she's not really doing things that are consistent with a broader vegan way of living. On the flip side, other people argued that if she raises her chickens in a way that's more humane, she's keeping factory-farmed chickens from a lifetime of suffering in cramped, horrid conditions. The common reaction to this was "yeah, but she's still killing animals." Sadly, the argument went on for awhile on the list, and we don't know if it ever got settled once and for all, but basically it broke down between vegans who preferred a harder-line definition of veganism and its roots in compassion, and vegans who felt that the woman deserved credit for her own veganism, and understanding for providing for her decidedly non-vegan family.

Though this is an extreme example, we've actually seen the whole question of defining veganism get heated and turn ugly. Similar fights break out over people who eat the occasional bit of dairy or eggs and proceed to call themselves "vegans." One way that people who are conflict-averse deal with this is by arguing that deciding who is and who isn't vegan is a waste of time, and that we should recognize all efforts as valid if they're actually in the direction of veganism. We have some limited sympathy for this approach, but as we see it, there's a danger in this kind of openness. If everything is potentially vegan—including being involved in the death of animals for human consumption—then veganism means almost nothing. What we mean is that if people who are eating milk and cheese call themselves "vegan," they destroy what veganism means. And for us, veganism means that you've made a commitment to reducing animal suffering and avoiding animal products to the greatest extent possible. No one needs dairy, eggs, leather, or wool except calves, chickens, cows, and sheep (in that order). Though we're ready to admit that there are areas of utter complexity when it comes to veganism and the avoidance of animal products (some of which we discussed in Chapter 1), there are areas that are completely straightforward and non-negotiable, and at least for us, these areas offer little flexibility if you call yourself a vegan.

For veganism as a movement of people who want to end animal cruelty and exploitation, diluting the message and meaning of veganism is dangerous. If people think of vegans as hypocritical idiots who are constantly decrying animal oppression while consuming the products of that oppression, our entire community takes a hit, and the protest that our choice represents becomes somewhat less understood. Veganism is as much an ethical protest as it is a way of living for one's own positive ends. If that protest is suddenly meaningless, we may feel better about what we're doing personally, but the visceral aspects of our statement as vegans in society gets muddied, lost, and misunderstood by the population at large. That's why we get fed up with people who aren't vegan calling themselves vegans.

vegan freak

Look at an analogous situation: many people think that vegetarians eat chicken and fish. When we were vegetarians, we grew utterly tired of being offered these animal products by people who thought they were being thoughtful and considerate of our diet. Part of that has to do with our not speaking up about our choices (like meek vegans, meek vegetarians suffer too), but another part of it has to do with the fact that there are "vegetarians" running around in the world who simply avoid red meat. This complicates life for vegetarians to no end. On top of it all, it makes the meat-eating "vegetarian" look like a fool. Fish do not grow out of the ground or on trees, nor do chickens.

We have no desire to be the vegan police, and given the reactions that we've seen elsewhere, we fear that we'll be read that way. Our goal isn't to tell you what to do with your life, or to tell anyone what to do. We'd prefer that people not eat chicken or fish, but if they're going to, that's their choice, and until they know better, we recognize that many people are going to make that choice. People will also continue to eat dairy products and eggs. Our point here is if you're going to eat animal products or be blatantly involved in the death of animals, **don't call yourself a vegan!**[13]

Some of you probably think we're being elitist, closing off veganism as our own private little club where only the most radical and marginal are members. This couldn't be further from the truth. We want everyone to embrace veganism. Our concern isn't to police the boundaries of our community for "bad" vegans who don't fit our mold of the "perfect vegan." Our concern is to have veganism *mean something* at the end of the day, rather than be a diluted "do whatever the hell you want" approach to preventing animal cruelty. Carol Adams goes as far as call-

---

13. Leather is more complex on this count; some people are wearing hand-me-downs or wearing their leather goods until they wear out. Though we think that wearing leather as a vegan sends the wrong message about veganism (and it is often one of the first things that people look for when they're scanning you for ethical inconsistencies) we realize that many vegans—especially new vegans—will likely still use their leather goods. There's a lot to be said for getting rid of your leather by giving it away/donating it/etc.(see Chapter 5).

ing these pseudo-vegetarians "saboteurs," and we think that's an apt description. There's little point in letting half-assed vegans sabotage the rest of us. (And if you're a pseudo-vegan reading this, do all of us in collective vegan freakdom a favor: stop calling yourself a vegan! We want you to be vegan, and we're here to help, but please be a vegan before calling yourself one!)

Approaching pseudo-veg*ns can be difficult. Some of these folks (particularly the pseudo-vegetarians) might actually not know any better. This might be hard to believe, but why not give them the benefit of the doubt? Pseudo-vegans probably *do* know better, but that doesn't mean that you should be too mean to them either. They may be even more deserving of your sympathy because their pseudo-veganism might be inspired by their desire to emulate some half-assed celebrity, and you gotta feel bad for anyone who wants to be like a celebrity.

The best route in either situation is careful conversation. Though we come down on pseduo-vegans pretty hard here, we suspect that few of them are reading this—after all, if they're pseudo-vegans, they're likely not so much into veganism that they'd bother reading a book on it. Our advice would be not to put anyone on the spot in front of others, but instead have a private conversation, or to offer to send the person literature or website links about veganism. On this count, Carol Adams suggests that you offer to send literature by Vegan Outreach, which is a fine suggestion. To that, we'd add that a quick look at Compassion Over Killing's eggscam.com should make it clear that eggs aren't vegan.

It can be surprisingly complex to deal with vegetarians of all stripes: the ex-vegan, the pseudo-vegan, and the hostile vegetarian. As with all interactions with hostile folks, it is important to remember the cardinal rule we stated earlier: many people become vegan because of the example of others. We're as sympathetic as anyone to reactions born of frustration, but those reactions won't get veganism any further ahead. Remember, you're representing something bigger here, even if you don't want to or didn't ask to, and the more diplomatic you can be, the better you advertise for veganism as a whole (and hopefully, create more vegans!). The real power in veganism is in its multiplier effect. Singly, we highlight some of the problems with animal exploitation, but if by example you can help more people go vegan, you can create a powerful multiplier effect that makes you a better proponent for compassion and ending animal cruelty.

Yes, freaky friends, dealing with the rest of the world isn't always easy, and we can't always please everyone, no matter how hard we might try. As you go through the various trials and tribulations you'll face as a vegan freak, you must remember the reasons that you've chosen veganism, why they matter, and why you need to stick with veganism despite the crap you'll get. Though you may be painted as an extremist radical who wants to challenge all that is right and good in the world, you must remember this is but a defensive mechanism on the part of your accusers. As long as omnivores can continue to consume without knowing or thinking about the conditions of exploitation involved in production, they can fool themselves into thinking their conscience is free and clear. Through your veganism, you remind them this transaction isn't so simple, and most omnivores want nothing less than to have to think about where their food comes from.

When people give you a hard time, or you're going through a rough spot, you must remember that you're living by your conscience, and living by one's conscience is never simple. On our blog (http://veganfreaks. org), Bob wrote the following entry about dealing with omnivores:

....some [omnivores] see fit to call me an extremist. Me? I'm just living by my conscience. If I'm to be true to my ethics, this is what I must do. Yes, it meant giving up blue cheese (which I loved, though which now seems gross), ice cream (though Soy Delicious rocks my socks), and cream in my coffee (soymilk works just fine, thanks) but these were the only choices to make since I couldn't in any way justify daily consumption of products that caused so very much suffering. Once I made myself think about it (which took some time, admittedly) there was no other way to go.

Bob knew, and couldn't un-know.

Regardless of how people view you, regardless of the personal problems that veganism might create, you must remember that you too know, and once you do, it becomes impossible to un-know.

This is something you cannot change for anyone.

Books and Other Sources Mentioned in This Chapter

- *The Pornography of Meat.* Carol, J. A. Continuum International Publishing Group. (2003).

- *Becoming Vegan: The Complete Guide to Adopting a Healthy Plant-Based Diet.* Davis, B., & Melina, V. Book Publishing Company (TN). (2000).

- *The Garden of Vegan: How it Vegan Again!.* Barnard, T., & Kramer, S. Arsenal Pulp Press. (2003).

TOAST

chapter four:
what DO vegans eat anyway?

This is a question that you are bound to hear frequently once you become vegan, because many people can't imagine what life would be like without meat, let alone dairy, eggs, and honey too. What's left to eat? Our usual answer to this question is everything else! Many meat-eaters have the misconception that when you become vegan, you're giving things up. We instead think of it as the opposite—when you become vegan, you open yourself up to a new variety of foods that you probably never would have tried or explored had you not gone vegan. You start to realize that being a vegan is about abundance, rather than a limited view of what makes a good dinner.

In this chapter, we'll go a little further into the definition of veganism, and tell you about some new foods you might want to try if you haven't already. In addition, we'll tell you about survival strategies so you don't go crazy in the grocery store, restaurants, or on the road. We'll also include some tips on living in non-vegan-friendly locales, like rural America. Finally, we'll discuss the possibilities of feeding vegan food to your pets.

What is Vegan?

Before we start telling you about the wonderful world of vegan cooking, we need to clarify what is vegan and what isn't. Though it should be clear by now, we'll say it again: vegans don't eat meat, dairy products, or eggs. But because the definition goes beyond that to reducing suffering and avoiding products from animals as much as possible, veganism becomes more than just the obvious. As a vegan, you'll most likely start to question not just the production of meat and dairy, but also the status of other beings like insects, and how animal products are used in food production in general. As we talked about in Chapters 2 and 3, people in Western societies are so removed from the process of food production that we have no idea where our food comes from, who grows it, makes it, or kills it, nor what is involved in any other process that gets it onto our dinner table. This chapter will shed light on some of these processes, helping you to decide what products you wish to use and which to avoid.

If you're ever bored and you feel like watching vegans attack one another mindlessly, pop on over to one of the forums in Appendix B and put up a post titled "IS HONEY VEGAN?"[1] (yeah, in all caps, they'll love you even more for that). Having said just that, you can sit back and watch as vegans go insane fighting over whether using honey is a big deal or not. If we happen to be members of the board you want to spam with honey questions, we'll be among the people there telling you honey isn't vegan. Okay, so kill us—we think you shouldn't exploit *any* life needlessly.

Most definitions of veganism that you can find agree with our assessment of honey as a non-vegan product. Many people, both vegan and non-vegan, often question why this is the case, because it is not as obviously egregious to animals as meat, dairy, or eggs. The basic answer is that in honey production, you are taking away a product that the bees normally produce for themselves and using it for your own needs, much like milk is taken from the cow for human use instead of being given to

1. Please don't really do this. You'll just be a pedantic pain in the ass.

her calf. While a bee is definitely different than a cow, it is an intelligent insect that is in the same phyla as lobsters and crabs (Arthropoda)[2]. Bees travel thousands of miles and visit millions of flowers to collect nectar to use in making honey, which then becomes their food for the winter. When commercial beekeepers take honey, they take all of it. Many bees are killed in the process, and many are lost over the winter. Bees have a central nervous system, and there is compelling evidence that they feel pain. Bottom line is, they're animals.

Another sweetener that poses a problem for vegans is refined (white) sugar. A lot of the sugar you'll find in the grocery store (like Domino) is not technically vegan, because refineries use bone char in the process of making sugar white. Bone char is the charcoal-like carbon left after incinerating animal bones[3]. The brown sugar from these same companies is only white sugar with molasses added, so it has the same problem. Raw sugars, beet sugar, and turbinado sugar are not bone char refined, and you can find companies that do not use bone char to refine their sugars, like Florida Crystals[4].

Besides trying one of these other types of sugars (which can be found in well-stocked grocery stores, co-ops, health food stores, and online), you might also want to try other sweeteners. Agave nectar is a really good substitute for honey, since it has a similar taste. You can also try maple syrup (the real stuff, preferably from Vermont), brown rice syrup, molasses, and stevia extract. How much you want to avoid sugar is up to you; we know many vegans who use vegan sugar and sweeteners at home, but might eat something with sugar of questionable origin on the road or in a processed food. Others try to avoid refined sugars completely, at least partially because sugar can make you fat (and definitely not phat).

---

2. http://www.vegetus.org/honey/honey.htm
3. http://www.sucrose.com/bonechar.html
4. http://www.vegfamily.com/articles/sugar.htm

But Beer is Vegan, Right?!

Now to the most important question—are beer and wine vegan? Even though you would think that beverages made from fermented plant products would be vegan, sigh, not all of them are. Fortunately, there are plenty of vegan beers and a few vegan wines out there. With beer, the problem is not necessarily with the ingredients per se (although some beers do contain dairy or honey), it is in how they are processed. After fermentation, beers go though a process called fining in which they are run through filtering agents to make them more clear. One of the traditional fining agents is called isinglass, which is made from the swim bladders of fish. Luckily, there are plenty of other filtering agents available, although some European breweries and many micro-breweries still use isinglass.

There is some good news, though: all German beers are vegan—it's been the law there since 1516—and many North American beers are as well. The major North American manufacturers and brands are all vegan (Anheuser-Busch (Bud, Michelob, Busch), Miller, Pabst Blue Ribbon, Rolling Rock), as well as other popular brands like Heineken, Sierra Nevada, Anchor Steam, Moosehead, Beck's, and Grolsch. So if you want to party it up with your PBR, you're good to go. Difficulty comes with microbrews (it varies greatly), British beers (many are not vegan), other European beers (besides German), as well as Mexican and Asian beers. If you ask us, it just plain sucks that they have to pollute otherwise perfectly good beer with dead animal remains.

Wine is yet more complicated. Like beer, wines are also fined through various ingredients, most of which are not vegan. Additionally, they may contain non-vegan ingredients. The fining agents and ingredients may include: eggs (albumen), dried blood, casein (dairy), chitin (from crustaceans), bone char, cochineal (insects), glyceryl monostearate, isinglass, lactose (dairy), gelatin, pepsin (from pork) and non-vegan sugars. Some manufacturers rely only on limestone, bentonite, silica gel, and other non-animal-derived fining agents. For example, most (but not all) organic wines are vegan (Frey Vineyards, Rutherford

Hill, etc.). There are also other vegan wines scattered across the globe. Your best bet is to look online or call the manufacturer to be sure (see resources below).

As we said in the introduction, how far you decide to go with your veganism is your choice alone. If you are okay with the fact that there are likely few animal products left in the beer when you drink it, then you can drink any brand. If you are unhappy that the beer is still processed with animal products and some remnants might remain in the bottle, then choose a purely vegan brand, as we do.

Most hard alcohol products are vegan, with a few exceptions to watch out for. The obvious is Irish Creme liquor. According to *Animal Ingredients A to Z*, most ports are fined using gelatin, and sherry is usually fined with animal products. Some vodkas may be filtered through bone char. Additionally, Campari is colored with cochineal.

Using *Animal Ingredients A to Z*, you can find out whether your favorite beer is vegan or not, since it contains a list of beers that manufacturers claim are vegan. There are also several lists on the internet that get updated when new information is found about different brands:

* PeTA: *http://www.peta.org*

* Vegan Porn: *no, it's not porn – see Appendix B; http://www.veganporn.com/booze.pl*

* Vegan beer list: *http://www.btinternet.com/~p.g.h/vegan_beer_list.htm*

* Vegan Vanguard: *http://www.veganvanguard.com/vegism/beer.html)*

* Vegans are from Mars: *vegan wine list - http://vegans.frommars.org/wine*

* Vegetarian Network Victoria: *mostly wines and hard alcohol - http://www.vnv.org.au/AlcoholByName.htm*

The best bet for your favorite brand is to call the manufacturer or visit their website, especially for microbrews that might not be on any list yet. Make sure you ask about not only ingredients, but processing agents as well. Then, go post your results somewhere on the Internet so that others can know (a good place to start are the forums on our website).

Having sorted out the drinks, now let's think about the main course...

What's for Dinner?

One day when Bob wore one of his vegan message shirts to class, one of his students raised her hand and said "You're a vegan? What do you eat? Like, apples and shit, or what?"

"Yes," he replied. "I eat only apples for three meals a day, every single day, 7 days a week. I alone support the economy of Washington State."

"Like, seriously?" the dumb student asked, drool running down her cheek, as she breathed through her mouth.

"Like, no," Bob replied.

So maybe Bob wasn't always the model vegan, but sometimes we just wear thin when we're asked such dumb questions, particularly when they come from gullible people. Nonetheless, vegans get asked what they eat all the time, partly because people are genuinely curious, and partly because people imagine that we've literally condemned ourselves to a diet of rice and beans.

For us, veganism has actually expanded the depth and variety of what we eat, and it isn't just rice and beans. When we first became vegan, we reinvigorated our love of cooking because we had so many new things to try. We started to realize how beautiful fresh produce could be, how good the herbs and spices smelled, and how delicious whole grains could taste – especially when their true tastes weren't being masked by dairy or eggs. Our cooking skills widened, and we started to enjoy ingredients and recipes beyond the veggie burger. Part of the challenge for the new vegan is that many are stuck in the mold of cooking what they probably grew up with; if you were a "typical American," dinner probably consisted of a big hunk of meat, a potato or rice dish, and vegetables on the side. If you spend your time just trying to replace that hunk of meat with another vegetable or meat substitute, things can get fairly boring. Even if you grew up eating non-Western foods, you might have only been exposed to a certain portion of them (i.e., the ones that had meat or other animal products). Another problem are the stereotypes about what vegans eat, and these stereotypes turn people off from even thinking about how to cook vegan.

If you visit a crappy middle-American restaurant, you're apt to believe that all vegetarians eat is pasta primavera and grilled vegetables. Oh, and of course, tofu. We've actually had people say to us "Wow, I could never be vegan. I really hate tofu."[5] To which we always want to respond "Wow, we could never be meat-eaters, we really hate meat." Seriously, though, people literally think we live on tofu and tofu alone, unless they own your average middle-American restaurant, in which case—if they even think about vegetarianism at all—they think we live on pasta primavera and grilled goddamn vegetables. Even when we were ovo-lacto vegetarians, there were few things more disgusting than looking at some overcooked linguine floating in the concoction of butter, cream, and salt that is often called "pasta primavera." Doesn't "primavera" mean "Spring" in Italian? What the hell is spring-like about something so damn fatty? And as for grilled vegetables, we love 'em, but for the love of god or whatever higher power you do or do not worship, how hard would it be for your average restaurant to come up with just ONE creative vegan dish? Point is, we eat more than pasta primavera, grilled vegetables, and tofu. And yeah, of course we think tofu is wonderful[6], and can be prepared in many delicious ways, but vegan cooking can be much more varied.

---

5. Most people who hate tofu have never had it prepared well. We've even heard of people who have tried eating it raw right out of the package. Are these people on crack?
6. We must mention that we've had delicious dinners consisting of grilled tofu, corn on the cob, and mashed potatoes with vegan gravy (thanks to inspiration from the Post Punk Kitchen), that do hit the spot sometimes. Plus we love Ma Po Tofu without the pork of course, and tofu scramble, and tofu ... you get the idea.

Rants about pasta aside, our first recommendation is to buy yourself a vegan cookbook that appeals to you based on the kinds of cuisines you like, how much time you can spend in the kitchen, and how much experimentation you like to do. This might seem like a common sense idea, but we know it's easy to forget about simple things when you're overwhelmed with a change in your diet. We recommend this even if you like to make up your own recipes, because it can spark a lot of new ideas for ingredients and preparations. You can even "borrow" techniques and ideas and weave them into your own creations. We've created a whole list of cookbooks in Appendix B and sorted them by category. You can also go online to find ever-changing databases of recipes, either submitted by readers (like http://vegweb.com) or from cooking gurus like the Post Punk Kitchen (http://www.theppk.com). If you have little or no experience with cooking, many cookbooks and websites have explanations of ingredients and techniques that will help get you off the ground. In reality, it isn't that hard to cook the basics well, and you don't even need much in the way of equipment to do it.

In these cookbooks, you'll find some traditional American-style recipes, but you'll also see examples of dishes that break the mold of the meat, potato, and vegetable platter that can help you envision new ways of conceptualizing your meals. You'll find dishes from cuisines around the world that you may not have tried before; even if you have grown up with them or been exposed to them before, you might find some new ideas. We are huge fans of Asian food, so we were attracted to recipes from China, Japan, Thailand, Vietnam, Korea, India, Pakistan, and Sri Lanka that we could make at home and then try in restaurants when given the chance[7]. Chinese greens and garlic, Indian dal, Thai curry, and Korean tofu bokum (just to mention a few) have become our favorites, despite having grown up with completely different foods and styles of eating. Of course, Asian food is not the only place you can find wonderful vegan dishes—there are recipes for Italian and other

---

7. See the section in this chapter on restaurants—there are some hidden ingredients like oyster sauce in Chinese food, fish sauce in Thai food, and ghee (butter) in Indian food that you should be aware of.

Mediterranean, Mexican and Latin American, French, African, Middle Eastern, and countless other cuisines available. You might even find options in a cuisine you've not considered in the past, like Ethiopian, which has delicious vegan dishes.

While you might be thrilled at the prospect of trying out this pano-ply of global cuisines, you might also be mumbling to yourself "...but what about all my old favorites? I'll miss them!" As we said earlier in the book, if you're living by your conscience and your principles, then the "sacrifice" is worth it. Plus, thanks to advances in food sci-ence, many of your old favorites can be veganized easily. Soymilk can be used in place of cow's milk in both baking and savory dishes (think mashed potatoes), as long as you don't buy the vanilla flavor (or choco-late. Could you imagine how nasty chocolate mashed potatoes would be?). Vegan margarine is available in place of butter, but read the label, because some margarine contains dairy in the form of whey. Alternately, you can use oil. Eggs can be easily replaced in baking with Ener-G® Egg Replacer (a powder that you add water to), or with tofu, bananas, applesauce, or ground flax seeds. Dairy yogurt can be replaced by soy yogurt. When we first became vegan, Jenna thought it was the end of making and eating baked goods, since we didn't know much about replacing everything with vegan versions. Thankfully, she was wrong. There are loads of great vegan baking recipes, and many non-vegan ones can be veganized easily. Many of the vegan baked goods we've tried taste as good as or even better than their original versions, and they fool even omnivores, who happily eat them up. If you don't tell them, they don't even come out with stupid comments about tofu, sticks, and twigs while they're eating.

If you miss your scrambled eggs for breakfast, try scrambled tofu. It's delicious[8]. Other breakfast items we can suggest are oatmeal, soy yogurt, cereal with soymilk, fresh fruit, smoothies, toast with vegan margarine, peanut, cashew, or almond butter, and/or jelly, homefries (a

---

8. See the cookbooks and online sources in Appendix B - many have specific recipes and suggestions for substitutes. You can also use tofu in place of egg for egg salad.

mix of regular and sweet potatoes is really good), vegan muffins, french toast, pancakes—basically whatever you're hungry for. Cold vegan pizza with Vegenaise®? Hey, whatever you're up for. And speaking of Vegenaise®, we have to mention that it makes a wonderful substitute for mayo. In addition to the obvious uses, a friend of ours suggests using this miraculous white substance for anything from freeing rings stuck on your finger to edible body paint. In short, the stuff rocks.

Cheese can be more challenging than replacing milk or eggs, because there are some really nasty cheese substitutes on the market, though there are brands that look, taste, and melt like real cheese (see grocery section of this chapter). There's even an entire cookbook (*The Ultimate Uncheese Cookbook* by Joanne Stepaniak) devoted to replacing your cheesy favorites. One thing that you'll find in replacing cheese is that nutritional yeast is your friend. Don't confuse this with the brown brewer's yeast you use to make beer or bread; nutritional yeast is a yellow flaky substance that smells and tastes cheesy. Many people use it in scrambled tofu, on popcorn (highly recommended), and in cheese substitutes. Plus, it's good for you since it's got lots of B vitamins. To make sure that you're getting all of these B-vitamins, we recommend only the RedStar® Vegetarian Support formula™. One more note on cheese—you'd be surprised how good a pizza without cheese tastes. Load it up with veggies (and even fake meats), and you're set.

If you think you'll miss ice cream, you'll be overjoyed to know that in the past few years, soy ice cream has come a *very* long way. Soy Delicious™ is one of our favorites, and receives nothing but high praise from all the vegans we know (and even non-vegans). Tofutti Cuties® are soy ice cream sandwiches to die for (but for which nothing has died). And if you're allergic to soy, there are tasty rice milk versions as well, like Rice Dream®. Rumor has it that there's even vegan soft serve out there somewhere. We dream of the day, however, when grocery stores have an entire aisle devoted to soy ice creams instead of dairy ice creams.

Fake meats have also gotten more popular, varied, and readily available in recent years. Read the labels to make sure they're vegan, since many of them contain eggs or dairy. You'll find your typical burger, hot dog, and lunch meat substitutes, but there's also a whole wonderful world out there based on wheat gluten or seitan, the protein from wheat. If you haven't tried seitan yet, we highly recommend it. You can find it refrigerated in vacuum-packed containers, frozen, or in cans. You can also make your own from wheat flour—there are recipes in many vegan cookbooks. Chinese cuisine has built amazing dishes based around various forms of wheat gluten and other substances that are meant to mimic beef, pork, chicken, ham, duck, and even shrimp, and that taste wonderful (and luckily not *too* much like the original).

Even though there are many substitutes for meat, eggs, and dairy on the market, you'd be doing yourself a favor if you tried more than just replacing what you already know. Once you start cooking without them, you'd be surprised how quickly your tastes change. We now find fake cheeses kind of disturbing because they taste too much like real cheese, even though we had cravings for it when first becoming vegan. As you can see from everything we've described in this section, you definitely won't go hungry. Though many people believe that veganism will limit your choices, we've actually found the opposite to be true.

Surviving the Grocery Store

As we just got done saying, there's plenty to eat as a vegan, but there's also plenty to watch out for. Along these lines, you can usually spot a fellow vegan in the grocery store by looking for someone who is standing in the aisle scrutinizing an ingredient label with a scrunched brow. You definitely know a vegan if you hear her muttering to herself something about dairy products or gelatin. Jenna has been known to spend at least 10 minutes in the bread aisle alone looking for a loaf of bread that didn't contain whey, milk, honey, or high fructose corn syrup, and that was also whole grain. The search usually ends with an exasperated "why do they have to put milk in bread?" and storming off without buying anything.

Going to a regular grocery store can be a mind-numbing and frustrating experience for a vegan, if for no other reason than you become amazed by the sheer amount of meat, processed foods, and things labeled "low-carb." On one hand, vegans have it better now than in the past. Soymilk, tofu, vegan veggie burgers, and other fake meat items are now readily available in most mainstream grocery stores, and produce sections have gotten bigger and more varied. On the other hand, processed foods and GMO foods are now more prevalent than ever, and people still think that carbohydrates are evil. Depending on where you live, it might also be hard to find some vegan specialty items.

On a trip through any grocery store, reading ingredient labels is a lesson in modern food science. As you read more and more labels, you become aware of how many chemicals we ingest every day and realize that most of them are a mystery; we have no idea how these foods are produced nor where the ingredients come from. As vegans, we also start to realize that many ingredients in processed foods are by-products of the meat industry, if not outright meat, dairy, or eggs. One of the upsides to this lesson is that we become more savvy consumers—we naturally think more about what we are putting in our bodies by looking at the ingredients and their nutritional content. As a result, we search for alternatives, perhaps leading us to a new-found appreciation for whole foods, as well as the support of companies and products that provide us with vegan versions of our favorite processed items. Of course, you can't avoid processed items completely, unless you're going to go out and grow your own soybeans and make your own tofu and soymilk. If, on the other hand, processed foods and chemicals don't bother you at all, you can find vegan versions of snack cakes, candy, and other junk in most grocery stores. Generally the cheapest stuff, these things contain crazy chemicals that will probably make you sterile, but if you're jonesin' for junk, this can give you your fix.

As a vegan, you have just about no choice but to read labels until you come to learn what brands are animal-free, so knowing how to read labels is an important part of surviving the grocery store. Recently, some label-makers have started making our job easier by highlighting common allergens in bold, and at the end of the list putting "contains

milk ingredients" or something similar. The most common dairy-de-
rived ingredients in processed food (apart from butter, yogurt, cheese,
buttermilk, etc.) include **casein** (milk protein, also caseinate or sodium
caseinate), **whey** (the liquid that separates from the solid curds when
making cheese and contains protein, fat, and sugars), and **lactose** (milk
sugar). These products show up in an amazing variety of processed
foods, since they are cheap and can add extra protein or another "nutritional" boost desired by the manufacturer. Whey and lactose are often
found in baked goods and breads—thus leading to Jenna's frustration
in the bread aisle—non-vegan margarine, and we've seen them in some
sports-drink mixes as well. Casein is responsible for one of the most
annoying and confusing parts about looking for vegan products—it
shows up in many items that are labeled as non-dairy! The typical
culprits are non-dairy creamers for coffee and non-dairy cheese. Yes,
you read correctly, *just because it says non-dairy does not mean it does not
contain ingredients derived from milk*. Apparently, casein helps soy and
rice cheeses melt like real cheese, so many companies include it. As an
aside, we really can't figure out why non-dairy cheese makers would go
to the trouble of making a soy cheese and then add milk products to
it. Is this meant to dupe vegans who aren't in the know? Is it just to
annoy us? Seriously, we don't get it. Seems like if you didn't care about
eating animal products, you'd just eat real cheese instead, but what do
we know? Anyway, the point is, you have to check the label carefully
because you can't assume that soy cheeses are vegan. There are alternatives like Vegan Gourmet™ and Tofutti Brand® cheeses that do not
contain casein which do melt fairly well, and taste surprisingly like real,
albeit processed, cheese. You can even find grated Parmesan substitutes,
or easily make your own.

There are other ingredients to watch out for besides the dairy derivatives and eggs. Gelatin, a by-product of the animal rendering process
(see Chapter 5 for a complete description), is most famously in Jello,
but also in marshmallows, candies, capsules and pharmaceuticals, and
miscellaneous other products. There are vegan ingredients that achieve
the same effect as gelatin, however, so you can find vegan marshmallows

and jello-type desserts. Honey, as we discussed earlier, is another popular ingredient in bread and baked goods, cereals, and snacks. Other animal ingredients include albumen (from eggs), glycerin (see chapter 5), and "natural flavors," which may be plant or animal based. (These "natural flavors" are why McDonald's french fries are not even vegetarian.) The source of the flavors do not have to be specified by the manufacturer, so they represent a gamble for vegans. Finally, some manufacturers use animal sources to derive vitamins, especially vitamins D, A, and B12. It is difficult to know the source of these vitamins without asking the manufacturer; your best bet is to go with products labeled vegan if you can find them. For instance, Silk® soymilk is completely vegan and is labeled as such, while other soymilks such as 8th Continent® still use lanolin as the source of their Vitamin D[9].

A basic rule of thumb is that if you haven't bought a product before and you haven't certified for yourself that it is vegan, check the ingredients carefully. Egg and dairy products show up in the strangest places. For example, we sometimes eat baked potato chips that we know are vegan, but recently we went to buy the BBQ flavor of the same kind and brand of baked chips, when we noticed it was not vegan (it contained both egg and dairy). Many veggie burgers contain cheese and/or egg, and you might find that some flavors or versions of a brand are vegan, while others are vegetarian. Gelatin also seems to be everywhere; we've even seen it listed as an ingredient in a package of sunflower seeds, which you would think would only contain sunflower seeds and salt.

If, like us, you aren't lucky enough to live somewhere that has an all-vegan convenience store like Food Fight! in your neighborhood, you end up doing a lot of shopping in a normal mainstream grocery store. In this case, you can eliminate a good portion of your frustration and label-checking if you spend lots of time in the produce department. We usually try to come up with a few new dishes to try each week that rely on fresh produce and whole grains. This way, we avoid eating too

---

9. http://www.vegparadise.com/news19.html

much processed food and we don't spend as much time or money at the grocery store. We also try to go to our local co-op as much as possible and highly recommend to others that they search for co-ops in their area (there is an online directory at http://www.cooperativegrocer.coop/coops/). Co-ops are basically owned by the people who shop there; members pay an annual fee and usually get a discount on groceries, plus the right to vote for board members who make the decisions that affect how the co-op is run. Co-ops usually carry a wide selection of vegan goods (as well as international foods, local foods, and "health" foods) and work with the local community that they serve in mind. They'll usually order single or bulk items on request as well, and can be good places to find large quantities of rice and other veggie cooking and baking staples. A final note on co-ops: don't let the self-involved Volvo-driving, NPR listening, middle-aged ex-hippie types scare you away from the good thing the co-op can be. Sure, they may have a holier-than-thou ethos about them as they pick through the organic arugula and talk about the latest production of the *Vagina Monologues,* but generally the co-op is a place that is friendly to vegans, and those ex-hippie types might even be vegans themselves.

Other places to try shopping are at international groceries that carry interesting new foods to try. Asian markets usually have the awesome fake meat products we discussed in the cooking section (either in cans, frozen, or fresh), noodles, tofu, fresh greens and other vegetables, and ingredients for sauces. Indian groceries have many kinds of lentils and dals, flours, and spices; Latin American and Caribbean groceries have tropical fruits and veggies, tortillas, sauces, and chile peppers galore. In addition, you might be able to find farmer's markets or fruit and vegetable stands, in both rural and urban areas. Buying produce at farmer's markets is excellent, because you are buying locally and in-season, and you can sometimes find specialty herbs and vegetables. These vegetables are usually very recently picked, so they taste significantly better than what you can get in the grocery store.

Then, there's always the internet. You can buy a wide variety of vegan items online, including some fresh and frozen food. We routinely buy all kinds of vegan goods online, mostly because we live in a county where there are more trees than people and where people call hunting, drinking beer, and driving ATVs (often at the same time) "fun." If you live somewhere rural like we do, online ordering might be your best bet. Alternately, get together with a few friends and put in a wholesale order at a whole foods supplier.

One last thing that you might want to investigate if you live in a rural area is a CSA, or community supported agriculture. You pay a flat fee to a farmer in the spring, and get fresh, usually organic vegetables delivered to you every week in the summer. CSAs are also available in some urban areas, but the costs are usually exorbitant.

Surviving the Restaurant

You already know that we live in a place where people love to hunt, so you can probably make the leap from that into imagining how much people around here love to eat meat, and when they go out, they like to eat LOTS of meat. As a result, going out to eat around here is pretty much a non-option for us, save a single Indian restaurant. Even if you're lucky enough to live in a town loaded with restaurants, there are plenty of things to watch out for when you go out to eat.

When you're stuck going to a regular, old American-style restaurant or even a bourgeois foodie-type place, you can probably ask for some kind of vegan entree, even if one isn't on the menu. If you're lucky, the chef or the ex-con in the kitchen cooking will make you something tolerable and vegan. If you're unlucky, they'll tell you that they can't accommodate you, and you'll be stuck sitting there munching on some iceberg lettuce while your friends eat their meals. When you know that you will be going some place where there might be limited vegan options, eat well ahead of time so that if you get there and there's nothing, you won't starve and get angry with everyone. Alternately, you can call ahead and ask if there's anything vegan. If the place is particularly "bou-

4. what DO vegans eat?

gie," you might even call ahead and ask them to prepare something for you, especially if you have a reservation. In any case, be completely and totally clear about what you can and cannot have as a vegan. Unless it is a vegetarian restaurant, they probably won't know what "vegan" even means, or will have some half-baked notion of what it is. Take care, or you could end up staring down a plate of pasta primavera.

Also, don't underestimate the power of a strategic lie. Tell the wait staff that you "cannot eat" fish, eggs, dairy, or meat or products that contain any of these things. They often take the "cannot eat" to mean that you are allergic, and restaurants take allergies seriously because they're afraid of being liable for your untimely death. Unfortunately, not many restaurants take vegetarians or vegans seriously, so you shouldn't feel too badly about lying to get your way. How far you decide to go is up to you. Saying that you "cannot have" animal products isn't technically a lie if you're vegan.

Should a restaurant go out of their way to be good to you, let them know you appreciated it. A quick letter helps, or even having a word with the manager. Conversely, if a restaurant treats you like hell, feeds you things that you explicitly tell them not to, and/or doesn't have much for vegans, you should also let them know. Politeness helps, even though you might really just want to scream at someone.

As we mentioned in the co-workers section in Chapter 3, "foreign" foods are your best bets for finding good vegan eats. Even so, ethnic cuisine is not automatically safe. Here we give a few quick warnings, grouped by cuisine:

Chinese: Dairy usually isn't a problem, but watch out for egg in soups. Dishes that seem vegan are often made with pork or chicken stocks. Ask if this is the case, and tell the server that you cannot have any chicken or pork stock in your food. Also watch for hidden meat, or meat popping up in places that you don't expect. The popular "Ma Po Tofu" often includes ground pork, but many restaurants will happily omit this if you ask. Chinese restaurants have usually been pretty flexible for us along these lines.

Indian: Watch for ghee (clarified butter), cream, and yogurt which show up in a variety of foods. In most Indian restaurants, you can assume that ghee is the cooking fat unless they tell you otherwise, and you should request that your food be made without it. Yogurt, cream, and cheese (paneer) are somewhat easier to avoid, as they're usually obvious in the descriptions of the dishes.

Italian: Ask if the sauces contain meat stock, meat, or cheese since you can never assume that they don't. This goes for pizza as well as pasta. Otherwise, you can usually get restaurants to make you a pasta dish or pizza without the cheese, but you'll probably have to remind them a million times.

Japanese: There's always vegan sushi, but watch out for stocks, as they often contain bonito (tuna). Fish hides in an infinite variety of places in Japanese cuisine. Your safest bet is to ask, or just stick to the vegan sushi.

Korean: Some kimchi is made with anchovies, some isn't. You can ask to be sure. Many dishes can be easily veganized in Korean restaurants, but don't assume that anything is vegan, even if it appears to be. Most Korean restaurants have been pretty cool about making us something vegan, even though the cuisine tends to be very animal-product centered on the whole.

Mexican: There's lots to watch out for with Mexican food (besides the gas). Lard is often used to prepare refried beans and tamale dough. Almost all corn tortillas are vegan, and many flour tortillas are as well, but you might ask to be sure. Watch out also for meat in bean dishes. You will need to specifically ask about meat and cheese in almost everything, but many dishes can be made vegan pretty easily if the people running the place are cool. Don't expect to get much of anything from that big chain that has a chili as its logo, however.

Thai and Vietnamese (Southeast Asian): Much Thai and Vietnamese food appears to be vegan, but is actually prepared with fish sauce. Make it clear that you cannot have fish or fish sauce, or you may end up with it, even in a dish that otherwise is vegan. Lots of Thai and

Vietnamese restaurants will happily oblige your request to go without fish sauce.

Regardless of the cuisine, there are things to watch out for, but once you learn the ins-and-outs, surviving restaurants isn't all that bad. You can find vegan Chinese food just about anywhere in a pinch, and if you're in a city, you can usually find something vegan without too much work. What can be challenging is traveling while vegan, and in the next section, we give you some tips for staying vegan on the road (or in the air, or on the train...you get the idea).

On the Road Again: Vegan Travel

Ah, the open road. Put the car in 6th gear, head down the interstate, and crank some music on the radio. The freedom ... the scenery ... and the ubiquitous fast food restaurant. Stopping for lunch on a road trip can be a quick lesson in why the standard American diet is so unhealthy, and why fast food joints are one of the reasons that factory farming is so prevalent, and the Costa Rican rain forest is disappearing so fast. Fast food is everywhere in the US—even in the most isolated places in the country—and there seems to be few alternatives. Whenever we travel, we can't help but think of the documentary *Super Size Me*. A thirty-day diet of nothing but fast food led Morgan Spurlock to damage his liver and gain 24 pounds; it definitely turns you off of even going into a fast food restaurant, unless you want to just go gawk in amazement of all the crap they have to eat and all the people that eat it (not to mention the fact that most of us likely used to chow down on it too).

If you're like us, you're never quite organized enough to think about packing a lunch when going on the road, and you are lucky if you leave within two or three hours of when you planned to leave. This means finding someplace to stop on the highway. We've driven across the country, and have found the offerings for vegans paltry. Unfortunately, this means that you might find yourself being forced to stop at a fast food place if nothing else is available. There are two fast food restaurants where you can reliably get something other than french fries: Subway and Taco Bell. We pretty much live on Subway subs when we travel.

You can get a Veggie Delight™ without cheese and mayo stacked with fresh veggies. Most breads at Subway are vegan except the obvious ones with cheese, and the wheat which contains honey. The only vegan condiments are mustard, oil and vinegar, and sweet onion sauce. Subs are also light enough so you don't feel like you're going to hurl when you get back into the car. The other option is Taco Bell. You can ask for a bean burrito without cheese and get a side of rice, which is now vegan. All the tortillas (corn and flour) and tortilla chips are vegan but chalupa shells are not; most of their sauces are vegan (including the guacamole). Check out the Veggie Fajita Wraps (make sure they don't have sour cream). The long-awaited veggie burgers now offered in some chains or some parts of the world have been disappointing, because like the BK Veggie™ Burger, they are vegetarian but not vegan (the burger contains egg and the bun contains dairy) (http://www.vrg.org). Plus, they're usually cooked on the same grill as the regular old deathburgers.

Most fast food salads seem to be loaded with meat or cheese (why do they have to ruin a perfectly good salad by throwing meat on it?) and rarely have vegan dressing options. Sometimes Italian and French dressings are vegan, but check the ingredients on the packet. If you get a french fry craving, Burger King and Wendy's are your best bet, since everyone else seems to use beef or chicken flavoring (e.g. McDonald's, possibly Arby's and Hardee's), or fries them in the same oil as chicken and fish. By the way, isn't it gross how you feel like you just used chapstick after eating fast food fries? Your whole mouth gets coated with grease. But we digress. As we mentioned above, you might want to keep your eyes open for a Chinese restaurant, since they'll most likely have a vegetable dish, or can make you something if you ask. Another possibility is a truck stop or other place with a salad bar. If you want a more complete list, go online to the Vegetarian Resource Group (www.vrg.org). They provide some updates on their site, and they sell guides to fast food restaurant ingredients.

You can definitely avoid fast food joints if you plan ahead and self-cater. Pack a salad, sandwich, or whatever else you can think of in a cooler. A lot of vegan cookbooks (Appendix B) have good suggestions for lunches or things you can easily take in the car with you. Stock up on snacks and beverages before you go—fruit, hummus, celery and carrots, nuts, veggie jerky, granola, pretzels, chips, other crunchy things, iced teas, little soymilk cartons, etc. If you want extra cool vegan snacks (assuming you can't find any locally where you live) put in an order ahead of time at Vegan Essentials (http://www.veganessentials.com) or Food Fight! (http://www.foodfightgrocery.com), both of which have an excellent array of crunchy snacks, sweet things (yes, vegan candy, chocolate, and cookies!), and energy-type bars. They also have vegan donuts and cereal-type bars, which are perfect for breakfast if you don't have time to go out or if you don't feel like searching for something vegan. Lastly, both retailers carry truly non-dairy creamers in small packets that you can take with you. We are die-hard coffee drinkers, and have found that soymilk is nearly impossible to find in coffee shops unless you're in a vegan-friendly town or larger city. If you think ahead or have time, you might be able to find small soymilk cartons at a grocery or convenience store. But pre-coffee, who can think that far ahead?

If you need to replenish your vegan snack and lunch supply along the way or if you get tired of Subway and Taco Bell, another option is going a little bit further off the highway to find a grocery store or co-op for a do-it-yourself meal. Some friends of ours take a co-op directory with them when they travel (available at http://www.cooperativegrocer. coop/coops/) so they can search out good places to stop in addition to finding good eats at the co-op; their reasoning is that if a town has a co-op, it probably has other cool things as well.

If you are traveling by plane, call the airline after you make your reservations to request a vegan meal, and again 24-48 hours before departure to confirm it. Take snacks with you on the plane, but stay away from fresh fruit if you're crossing a border or going to an agriculturally sensitive place like Hawaii—they'll most likely confiscate it, you vegan terrorist.

When you're at your destination—unless you're in, say, South Da-kota—things get a little easier (and more healthy) because you'll have a wider array of restaurants to choose from. If you're going to a large city, search online before you go for one of the many vegetarian dining guides available (some are printed by smaller presses, or groups that live in the city, and may be particularly helpful). Or, you can search one of the online lists of vegetarian and vegan restaurants around the world. These lists are not exhaustive, since there may be more veggie-friendly restaurants in the area that didn't make it to the list, but they can give you some reliable information on good options. Additionally, check is-sues of magazines like *Herbivore* and *VegNews* for restaurant reviews and lists. Here are a few places you can start your search:

* *http://www.happycow.net/*

* *http://www.vegguide.org/*

* *http://www.vrg.org/restaurant/index.htm*

* *http://www.vegdining.com/Home.cfm*

* *http://www.vegeats.com/*

Individual cities often have their own lists, so do a Google search to find out. And here we repeat our restaurant mantra once more: if you're having trouble finding vegan options, again try to find a Chinese, Indian, or other international restaurant that will likely have one or two vegetable dishes. There's always pizza and pasta as well. Many pizza places will make you a pizza without cheese on request (unless you're extremely lucky to find a vegan cheese pizza), even though they'll prob-ably look at you funny. With pasta and cheeseless pizza, however, you need to make sure the sauce is vegan; some places add cheese and/or meat to the sauce, as we noted above. In places like this, ask for a base of olive oil and garlic instead.

We have a hard time getting up and getting out the door before places start serving lunch, but when we have been up for it, we've found breakfast to be one of the harder meals for dining out, especially if you're not lucky enough to be in an area that has a veg*n cafe that serves tofu scramble. (And no, Dunkin Donuts and Krispy Kreme are not vegan.) You can bring fruit, vegan donuts or bars with you as we already mentioned, or if you're in a place with access to hot water, instant oatmeal. You might find yourself self-catering at a grocery strore or co-op, or searching out a bagel place to get a bagel with peanut butter, but beware of bagels with egg or honey. Diners and cafes often have oatmeal and fruit available; you might also want to ask if the homefries are cooked with butter or bacon fat. More often than not, homefries are cooked on the same grill as meats too, so you can sometimes end up with stray bacon bits in your fries.

If you're going to a foreign country and don't speak the language or don't speak it well, find out how to say "I'm a vegan" in the language and practice it. It is best to learn a phrase that also says you don't eat eggs and dairy. The International Vegetarian Union (http://www.ivu.org) has a list of useful vegetarian phrases in an impressive number of different languages, as well as other helpful travel resources. You might also want to make yourself a bilingual list of things that you do and do not eat with the help of a phrase book or dictionary, so that you can watch out for these items on menus. When traveling internationally, watch for small open-air markets which may have wonderful produce to try. Then again, these open air markets also usually have pretty smelly butchers and fish markets, so you can decide if you can stomach it or not. Similarly, in North America, you can also keep an eye out for farmer's markets and roadside stands.

Planning ahead when you travel can make your experience much more enjoyable. One more tip is to buy a set of refillable bottles for your favorite cruelty-free toiletries, so you don't have to use the ones that your hotel or host provides. Finally, look for vegan-friendly businesses when you travel and support them. Though they're a bit too dainty for our tastes, if you enjoy staying at bed and breakfasts, there are many that serve veg*n food and are veg*n owned.

Here's a summary of the basic list of things you might want to bring with you on a trip:

* vegan snacks: *crunchy/salty and sweet - you never know what you might crave!*
* self-catered lunch
* fresh fruit: *surprisingly hard to find on the road; don't take on international travel*
* vegan coffee creamer packets and/or soymilk cartons
* quick breakfast options: *vegan donuts or cereal bars; instant oatmeal*
* vegan mints
* refillable travel-size bottles for toiletries
* veg dining guide: *or list of veg-friendly restaurants from internet*
* co-op directory: *http://www.cooperativegrocer.coop/coops/*
* for international travel: *a card that says "I'm a vegan" in whatever language is spoken, as well as a list of items that you do and do not eat.*

This should cover most of the basics for vegan eatin'. At this point, you should have some ideas about new foods to try, how to survive the grocery store, restaurants, and how to travel. Some of these tips and ideas might seem like common sense, but believe it or not, you can get so caught up with all of the other aspects of veganism that even the easy stuff can slip through the cracks, particularly when you're a new vegan. Of course, what we have to say is never the final word. By way of being shamelessly self-promotional one more time, if you have good tips, ideas, or suggestions, you should visit our website and inform other readers. This way, the word gets out there a bit further.

So, we've pretty much dealt with what *you* should eat, but there's one final bit that we'd feel remiss if we didn't discuss. Namely, can you make your pets vegan? When most people hear this idea, they think it is insane. Aren't dogs carnivores? Don't dogs and cats literally *need* meat to live? When we first heard of the idea of vegan pets, we thought it was insane, but then we gave it some more thought, read up on it, and were pleasantly surprised by how possible it seemed. In the next section, we discuss veganizing your pets, and why we think it is something worth considering very seriously.

Is Your Dog a Vegan?

When relatively hostile people find out that you're a vegan, they dig for ethical inconsistencies. It seems a lot of people imagine that we vegans live like monks who've sworn themselves to a life of what omnivores see as culinary poverty—having given up McNuggets and burgers and other pillars of the fat-inducing standard American diet, they imagine that we somehow have the ethical wherewithal to eat only salad and tofu for the rest of our lives. As we discussed in Chapter 3, many omnivores feel judged simply by the presence of vegans, forget about even talking the politics of veganism. We remind them that they're eating dead things. For some people that's an uncomfortable realization, and one that they'll fight at all costs.

If omnivores do find ethical inconsistencies, they feel it gives them license to declare us hypocrites and acquit themselves. Any vegan reading this has been at one time or another searched up and down for leather by a grumpy omnivore, or quizzed on the extent of one's veganism. If you're able to overcome these challenges and you're up against a particularly trenchant omnivore, you might notice a point in the conversation when a quick smile crosses their face and they ask "okay, then, mr. fancy-pants vegan activist weirdo freak, what the hell do you feed your dog if you object so strongly to killing animals for food?"

When we first became vegans, this was the omnivore trump card. We had no choice but to say "yeah, well….umm, yeah, we feed our dog regular dog food." It just never even occurred to us that there was another option. We used to go to the food store and buy a bag of dog food, despite the fact that it was made with ground up bits of turkey or chicken or even lamb, well, because that's what dogs eat. And cats? They're definitely carnivores—just look at their teeth! But then we started thinking that these are the same arguments that people use to defend eating meat: humans have been eating animals "forever," we need meat to survive and be healthy, and it's what we're "supposed to do." Are cats and dogs in the same position as humans in this case? Could they be happy and healthy on a vegan diet?

In short, the answer is yes. If you have a dog or cat, you must run out now and go get Jed Gillen's excellent book *Obligate Carnivore: Cats, Dogs, and What it Really Means to be Vegan.* Gillen's book approaches the question of vegan pets with a balance of sensitivity and humor. Upon reading the book, we realized that our dog was already a canine garbage disposal for our vegan scraps. He eats things that we've never seen dogs eat – things like bananas, grapes, tofu, oranges, and even dried chile peppers. Why not vegan dog food? Gillen's book got us thinking about making our voracious lab a vegan, especially after he detailed some of what ends up in pet food. Disgustingly, your cat or dog may be turned into an unwitting cannibal, since shelter-killed animals (and traces of the drugs used to kill them) sometimes end up in pet food. Basically, cats and dogs eat the leftovers of the slaughter industry, including animals that were sick or "downed" at the time of slaughter. Pet food may also contain rotten meat from grocery stores and fast food joints, road kill, and of course, euthanized pets. Ever wonder why your cat pukes so much? It might just be the odd assortment of chemicals and rotten meat that he's eating.

And as to the question of whether or not a vegan diet is healthy for dogs and cats, Gillen provides plenty of arguments describing why cats and dogs who live in our homes do not need to eat meat. Like humans, as long as cats and dogs get all the essential nutrients they need, they will be healthy. If we are supplying them with a balanced kibble or recipe that contains synthesized or plant-based taurine, arachidonic acid, and other nutrients, we are giving them everything they need. Cats need a little extra care than dogs to get the right nutrients (especially because they are picky eaters), and Gillen includes a special section on cats with urinary-tract problems that you need to pay attention to if your cat, like ours, has had difficulties in this area.

It might seem like a drag to read a whole book on cats, dogs, and veganism, but Gillen's writing is engaging. He's conversational and funny, and you feel like you get to know him. The balance of humor and seriousness that he brings to the work draws you in, and best of all, it gets you to think seriously about what it really does mean to be a vegan, and how much you really want to contribute to an industry that you're likely opposed to. Most vegans we know who have pets love them like they were their own children (or more so, in some cases). They play with them, go for walks with them, take them to work, post pictures of them on the internet, and let them lick their faces without question (which may not be so wise if the pets were just licking certain parts of themselves). So if people love their pets so much, why do they continue to feed them animal products while they try to avoid them as much as possible?

After reading Gillen's book, we switched our lab over to Evolution Vegan Kibble[10] and we haven't looked back. This food is a bit more pricey than your conventional death-chow, but the dog loves it and after having eaten pretty much only this for the last year (plus the occasional hunk of tofu that we drop on the floor when cooking) he's in excellent health. He's active, full of energy, and always ready to play—sometimes too ready to play! On top of it all, we feel better feeding him food that is entirely vegetable-based. His food is certain to exclude animal shelter kills and rotten meat, and it has all the nutrients that he needs to be healthy and happy. If you have companion animals and are thinking of making them vegans too, check out Gillen's book. He gives you all the data that you need to make a considered and intelligent decision about whether your companion animal should be a vegan or not.

People who know us know our dog—he's a big part of our lives— and when they hear that he's a vegan too, they're usually shocked because he is "so healthy and has so much energy." Not only have we cut out the omnivore trump card, but we also provide concrete evidence to the doubters out there that both humans and dogs can be healthy as vegans. Ethical inconsistencies be gone!

---

10. See Appendix B for places where you can buy vegan dog and cat food online.

And Finally....

Some people view veganism as a closing off of options, but for us, it has meant much more than that. Against even our own expectations, veganism has opened us up to a new variety of foods and changed our experience with food for the better. Casting animal products out of our life, we filled the space with new and different kinds of foods, different cooking techniques, and new approaches to eating. In sum, there's plenty to eat as a vegan. Provided you don't eat just potato chips and cheeseless pizza, you can do just fine on a vegan diet, and beyond that, you can probably thrive. The key, as with any diet, is to eat a variety of things.

Though the most immediate and practical dimension of veganism is what we do and do not eat, ethical veganism is about more than this. Most ethical vegans seek to reduce the use of animal products to the greatest extent possible, which includes what we wear. In the next chapter, we discuss some basics of vegan fashion, and the ever-timely question of what to do with all that old leather that you probably own!

Books and Other Sources Mentioned in this Chapter

- Why Honey Is Not Vegan: *http://www.vegetus.org/honey/honey.htm*

- Vegan Sugars: *http://www.vegfamily.com/articles/sugar.htm*

- Bone Char: *http://www.sucrose.com/bonechar.html*

- Vegetarian Resource Group: *http://www.vrg.org*

- International Vegetarian Union: *http://www.ivu.org*

- *Animal Ingredients A to Z : Third Edition.* E.G. Smith Collective. AK Press. (2004).

- *Meatless Meals for Working People: Quick and Easy Vegetarian Recipes (Meatless Meals for Working People).* Wasserman, D., & Stahler, C. Vegetarian Resource Group. (2001).

- *Obligate Carnivore: Cats, Dogs, and What it Really Means to be Vegan.* Gillen, J. Steinhoist Books. (2003).

chapter five:
fur is dead. and leather too. and wool.

Veganism is not just about food. Ethical veganism is also about reducing suffering to the greatest extent possible, and reducing our reliance on animal products as much as possible. As vegans, we become much more knowledgeable consumers because our desire to live our ethics means we have to learn about ingredients, materials, and methods of production. As we said in Chapter 1, deciding what to buy based on this knowledge isn't meant to be a crippling exercise—you need to figure out what is feasible and reasonable for you to do. That said, there are a lot of alternatives available to the animal products we've become accustomed to, and if you know what to look for and where to look, you can easily be on your way to becoming less reliant on animal products.

For better or worse, if you're a vegan and people know it, you're representing veganism as a whole. Yes, this sucks. No, it isn't fair. And of course you never asked to be the spokesperson for an entire movement, but given the way that most people function and the way they make logical leaps, this is how you'll be considered. Most people won't give vegans the benefit of the doubt. They won't bother to find another vegan if one they met previously was a fool, or illogical, or even contradictory. And for this reason, wearing wool, silk, fur, leather, or down simply sends the wrong message about veganism and the commitment you've made to it. Leather-wearing vegans are walking contradictions; on the one hand, they argue that we need to stop exploiting animals, but on the other, they're wearing the skin of a dead animal. Many people will read this as a vegan who is lax in their principles, or they'll read it as someone who is just simply a hypocrite. On the flip side, if you can wear clothes that don't come at the cost of animal exploitation, you can send a powerful message about veganism and your commitment to it. In addition, you show that you can be fashionable without resorting to animal exploitation. You don't need the flesh, fur, or feathers of another animal to make you look cool or to stay warm in the winter, particularly when there are options that are easier than ever to find.

At the outset, it's completely obvious why a product like leather is not vegan, since it is a product of the meat and dairy industries (or some say vice versa). Despite this, many people assume that wool isn't so bad, since you don't have to kill the sheep to get it. Like dairy cows, however, old sheep whose wool-producing days are over are killed for meat. The shearing process can cause injury to the sheep, and leaves them exposed to both heat and cold. Like the pigs we described in Chapter 2, farmers castrate the sheep, dock their tails, and clip their ears without anesthetic. The castration process is particularly painful. For many sheep, a castration band is wrapped around the scrotum until it loses its blood supply and falls off[1]. Merino Sheep are also bred to have a great deal of skin[2]. Why? Because more skin means more available surface for wool growth. These extra skin folds are susceptible to infestation by flies and maggots, to which farmers respond by cutting off strips of skin from the hindquarters of live animals[3].

At this point, we probably don't need to explain why fur is so hideously torturous, but in case you need convincing, we'll give you a few quick and gruesome facts. Many fur animals are now raised in fur mills where they cannot leave their cages for their entire lives. As a result,

---

1. Holy hell, writing that sentence just made me wince! -Bob
2. Tom Regan, *Empty Cages*
3. http://www.peta.org/mc/factsheet_display.asp?ID=55

they suffer from what are essentially "psychotic" conditions from their confinement and spend significant proportions of their lives pacing in their cages. When animals are killed, they are often gassed or anally electrocuted. In some cases where the slaughter was not effective, animals are actually skinned alive, or find themselves waking up from the initial shock of slaughter while being skinned. On top of all of this, the Humane Society of the United States estimates that some two million dogs and cats are stripped of their fur in China and other Southeast Asian countries each year[4]. Much of this fur ends up on stuffed animals, as trim on parkas, and even full-length coats. Think you won't consume any of this because you don't live in China? Fat chance. Much of what is produced in China is exported throughout the world, including Asia, Europe, and North America.

In the end, there's just no point in wearing leather, wool, fur, or down. Why try to create moral excuses and justifications for these products when you know better?

But What Do I Do With the Old Leather?

Still, even if you know better, what to do with old leather, wool, and other animal-based stuff is complicated by a number of factors. When we first became vegans, we did a quick inventory of our clothing and found lots of leather shoes and belts, wool sweaters, a down comforter and pillows, and down and wool coats, which we thought were absolutely necessary to survive our winters here where the temperature routinely drops below 0 degrees F. Since we didn't have the money to replace everything right away, we had to take a triage approach. We decided to start with our shoes and belts, since they were the most visible and said the most about our public image as vegans. The last items to be replaced were our pillows and comforter, since they were only visible to us and were also expensive.

When it comes to what to do with your leather, wool, down, and silk, there are basically three options: use it until it wears out (and ex-

---

4. Tom Regan, *Empty Cages*

plain to people in the meantime why you are wearing it), give it away or sell it, or throw it out. Some see it as a waste to throw it away or get rid of it, especially if it is still usable. Others want to replace it as soon as possible and use it as an excuse to go on a shopping spree. A common sense approach that many fellow vegans choose is to donate items (or if they're really new, sell them), because that way they will live out their useful lives with someone else. Then, when they have the money, they can replace the items with vegan versions.

In deciding what is right for you, you need to take into consideration how you want to represent veganism and live by your ethics. Choosing to wear leather shoes might water-down what it means to be vegan, but not all of us have extra cash lying around to buy new things right away, even though there are plenty of cheap vegan shoes at places like Payless. If you have the money, the question becomes easier, but you might still be holding onto things for sentimental reasons. We know that your absolutely favorite sweater might be wool, but remember that by choosing to live without it, you're showing that you don't need wool to survive, that vegans can live happily and fashionably without animal products, and that you are being consistent in your beliefs. Plus, your sweater will wear out eventually, so why not replace it sooner rather than later? It can become someone's else's favorite thrift store find.

Our advice is simple: give it away if you can and replace it as soon as possible. If you can't get rid of it all at once, remember that veganism is about doing your best, not about perfection.

Pleather is Punk

Once you do decide to get vegan goods, you need to figure out what items can replace what you have, and where to find them. Remember the vegan in the grocery store looking at labels? You can also spot your fellow vegan in the shoe store doing a happy dance upon finding the words "all man-made materials." Yep, those magical words tell you your shoes aren't leather. If you're looking to save some dough, bones, skins or whatever it is you cool kids are calling money these days you can find cheap vegan shoes at chain stores like Payless. Otherwise, higher-end chain stores will mostly be leather, but might have the rare vegan find—you won't know until you look.

If you want to remove the guess-work and searching, there are vegan shoe stores out there, like MooShoes in New York and OTSU in San Francisco. Luckily for those of us who live far from these magical vegan places, you can order online. In fact, if you're not afraid of ordering shoes online without trying them on, you can find tons of vegan shoes on the Internet, at Alternative Outfitters, Vegan Essentials, Pangea, Earth Shoes, and more. Besides all-vegan stores (for this whole section, check the resources we list in Appendix B), you can also find a wide range of non-leather shoes on Zappos.com (and they'll get them to your door amazingly fast). Still, we recommend that you support vegan retailers first, as they're trying to make a living at creating a more cruelty-free world.

There are vegan versions of all your must-have types of shoes, including sandals, running shoes, and hiking boots. Some of the more expensive vegan shoes use material that's much stronger than the cheap vegan shoes, so they do tend to last longer. Some materials also look a lot like leather, which can be a good or a bad thing, depending on your opinion. Many people want to get away from the look of leather because it creates a new sense of what's fashionable, rather than trying to look like dead cow. Others like to make a statement that you can have the look of leather without killing anything. Bob, for example, loves his 14-hole steel-toed pleather boots. They simply kick ass.

Like shoes, the cheaper versions of handbags and belts also tend to be non-leather. Many of the vegan shoe stores and online shops we listed above also carry bags and belts. We've also found quite a few small manufacturers online that make their own line of (usually) handmade vegan bags, like Queen Bee Creations (vinyl bags) and M. Avery Designs (cloth bags). Jenna can gush for anyone who's interested about how really fucking cool her Queen Bee truckette is.

Replacing down and wool is easy, since cotton and synthetic fibers abound. Winter coats, however, have provided us with one of the toughest challenges, because it's colder than all get out (as Jenna likes to say) where we live. Every coat that can provide warmth in temperatures below -15 F seems to be down. Down is very warm—after all, that's why the goose needs it! Fleece, on the other hand, is a gift from the gods of synthetic materials that is meant to save you from the cold. You can find some fairly heavy-duty coats that can hold their own in the winter that are either made from fleece or that have a fleece layer. If they don't hold up, you can always add a layer of fleece. Check for brands like Columbia, Mountain Hard Wear, and North Face.

One last place you can look for clothing items are thrift stores, especially if you have a keen eye. Thrift stores can be good because they are cheap and they have a wide array of items, not to mention the fact that they are providing an outlet so we can reuse items rather than throw them away. Sarah Kramer, in the *The Garden of Vegan* and *Herbivore* magazine talks a lot about being a thrift store junkie, if you're interested in hearing more about the wonders of the thrift store. Personally, we dig the thrift store ethos, but the key to thrift store success is getting there before all the trendy emo kids do.

It may seem like a pain at first to find vegan clothing and accessories and to replace what you have. Believe us, we know how frustrating it can be when you're looking for a non-wool sweater and it seems like everything you find is wool. But in time you start to learn about places where you can consistently find items you like, and it gets easier. Who knows—maybe you'll be inspired to design an all-vegan clothing line or start your own vegan store (any fashion designers out there?). In the end, you'll find that you walk taller in your new vegan gear. It gives you confidence and a sense of well-being to know that no animals were killed for your fashion.

Now that we've dealt with not wearing dead animals, we need to talk about one last place where animal products end up—in cosmetics and other personal care items.

Vegan Cosmetics and Toiletries

Animal products have a tendency to show up in places where we least expect them, and in things that we rely on everyday: soap, deodorant, medicines, makeup, lip balm, shaving cream, lotion, and many other drugstore items. Animal ingredients are cheap and plentiful, and are used without question by many large companies who also test their products on animals. They are also harder to identify than the dairy and egg-derivatives in grocery items, since many are listed only by their chemical name. You might think that searching the ingredient list of not only your groceries but also your toiletries is a major pain in the ass. Perhaps you'll conclude after skimming enough ingredient lists that this level of vigilance is unnecessary, but we'd like to convince you otherwise. Since there are so many non-animal alternatives, it is relatively easy to find products that are vegan-friendly and cruelty-free. And after you learn about the processes used to get animal products into most cosmetics and toiletries, you'll probably want to seek out animal-free options.

Understanding the rendering process is essential for understanding why it's necessary for vegans to be concerned about what's in the products they use. Once animals are slaughtered, all the leftover parts (bones, ligaments, hooves, brains, spinal columns, eyeballs, intestines, and other random parts) are sent off to a rendering plant, along with euthanized pets from shelters, horses, road kill, and spoiled meat from the grocery store. (We're not making this up.[5]) The hooves and ligaments go into making gelatin, which shows up in Jello, pharmaceuticals (capsules), gummy candies, marshmallows, and film. Other bits are all boiled together in a big, nasty soup. What sinks to the bottom is what goes into cat and dog food, and is also fed back to livestock (ever wonder where mad cow came from?). What floats to the top of the soup gets made into cosmetics, soaps, shaving cream, shampoo, pharmaceuticals, crayons, candles, and even toothpaste. Pretty disgusting, isn't it? Now,

---

5. Howard Lyman, *Mad Cowboy.*

do you really want to be brushing your teeth with that, or rubbing it on yourself as lotion?

Luckily, there are many non-animal-based equivalents to the things that come out of the rendering process. Unfortunately, animal-based products are cheap and readily available because of the billions of animals slaughtered every year. It's a huge business, and therefore these products show up in just about every product imaginable in your local drug store or grocery store.

The best way to find out about insidious animal ingredients is to get a copy of a book like *Animal Ingredients A to Z* or *PeTA's Shopping Guide for Caring Consumers*[6], which also has a list of companies that do and do not test on animals. Both books are cheap and extremely useful.

In the absence of those books, we'll list some of the more common ingredients to watch out for:

• **Glycerin:** usually made out of animal fats left after making soaps. Ever see *Fight Club?* Same principle applies here. Glycerin shows up in lotions, shampoos and conditioners, soaps and body washes, cosmetics, tattoo ink, and toothpaste. There is a plant-based form of glycerin, and some companies will list its source. If it's not labeled, chances are at least some of it is animal-based.

• **Lanolin:** comes from sheep's wool, and according to PeTA's guide, is a known allergen. This product is in many lotions and body washes, as well as lip balm and other skin-care products. Vegetable oils can serve the same function without harming sheep.

• **Stearic acid:** (and its derivatives; look for the prefix stearo-) comes from the stuff that floats to the top during rendering, and also from the stomachs of slaughtered animals. Yuck. This one is in the same kinds of products: shaving cream, cosmetics, deodorants, hairspray, and even some food and chewing gum. You can get stearic acid from plants (like coconuts, for instance), but since rendering is such a big business and

---

6. Also available online at http://www.caringconsumer.com.

the products are so cheap, many companies will just use the animal-based versions.

Those are the three most insidious products that we've come across, since they seem to be in just about everything. There are plenty of others to watch out for, like the already mentioned gelatin, beeswax, polysorbates, alpha-hydroxy acid, and ingredients like keratin and other proteins, found in skin-care products, and shampoos and conditioners. Get one of the guides to familiarize yourself with the types of ingredients to watch out for.

If you're ever not sure about whether the glycerin or stearic acid in your favorite beauty product or toothpaste is from an animal source or not, call the company that manufactures it. That way you'll be sure, and you'll also be letting the company know that there are people out there who are concerned about this type of thing and who won't want to buy their product if it has animal bits in it. Any step away from society's reliance on animals is a good one. It's probably best to stay away from the large manufacturers anyway, since most of them test on animals.

At this point you might be wondering how you can avoid all of these ingredients if they're so very common. One of the easiest ways that we've found to get vegan beauty products is to shop online at a place like Vegan Essentials (http://www.veganessentials.com; see Appendix B for other sites as well). They do the label reading for you, so you know that everything they sell on their site is vegan (they even look out for honey and beeswax and carmine/cochineal, which is made from crushed-up insects.) Plus, you can buy shampoo, bath gel, soap, makeup, lip balm, lotion, skin cleansers, deodorant, shaving cream, etc. all in one place (along with some awesome snacks and vegan shoes! Can you tell that we couldn't live without Vegan Essentials? And they didn't even pay us to say this!). There are also lots of small manufacturers that produce vegan products and sell them online, such as Dirty Kitty Soap Works or Crazy Rumors lip balm (see Appendix B for complete list of sources and web addresses). A lot of these places are vegan-owned as well, so they are great options if you find products you like. Always support other vegans when you can!

Locally, you will probably be able to find brands like Kiss My Face, which makes facial care products, lotion, deodorant, soap and bath gel, and other goodies. JASON is another easy to find brand. In addition, Tom's of Maine, which makes toothpaste and mouthwash mostly, but also deodorant, shampoos, and soaps, can be found pretty easily in grocery stores or drug stores, even in the redneck rurality that we live in. Your local co-op or health food store might also have a nice selection of vegan products, but you still want to read the label to be sure. Beware that some "natural" products—even in some brands we mention above—contain lanolin, beeswax, and honey. We cringe when we hear of Burt's Bees described as a cruelty-free company.

If you're wondering whether these products are more expensive, the truth is that they probably do cost a little more than you're used to paying. What we've found, however, is that these products tend to last a lot longer because they are higher quality. We've had some of these products last for months, with frequent use. We've found that we end up either spending the same amount of money or even saving money in the end. Most importantly, you won't be supporting companies that either test on animals or use animal products. Overall, this is a winning deal.

If you're a product junkie like Jenna or if you are into higher-end hair-care and beauty products, check out Aveda (http://www.aveda.com), which does not test on animals. Aveda says their products are "people tested," and they have also told us—repeatedly—that they do not use animal sources for their glycerin, stearic acid, etc. even though their labels might not be clear as to the source (some list the source, some don't). They do use beeswax and honey in a few of their products, so watch for those.

Going to a salon that uses Aveda products is also a way to make sure that when you get your hair cut or colored, you're not using animal products. Of course if you're like us and you don't live anywhere near a salon that carries Aveda, you don't have much choice as to the products they use in your hair, but you can bring your own products if you want. The final option is to cut your own hair or get someone you know to do it, although Jenna refuses to cut Bob's hair because she really, tragically fucked up someone's haircut in the past. She recommends you not try to cut hair after a few beers.

Yet another way to avoid questions as to whether there are animal products in your personal care items is to make your own. If this appeals to you, check out books like *How it all Vegan* and *The Garden of Vegan*. Both of these are cookbooks, but they also have sections on natural beauty products that are easy to make, as well as very useful sections on the many uses of vinegar and baking soda.

The goal is to reduce your reliance on animal-based products, since unfortunately it's nearly impossible to be 100% animal-free. If you accidentally buy a product that you later find out to have an animal ingredient in it, return it, throw it out and buy a new one, give it away, or learn from your newfound knowledge and buy something else next time. Think about how happy you'll be knowing that you just washed your face and brushed your teeth with an entirely plant-based product.

Don't Read This Section if You're Under 18

Titling any section like that virtually guarantees that those under 18 will read it, but what can we do? Were Bob under 18 and not the author of this book, this section would probably be the first thing that he'd have read. Anyway, in this section, we talk about yet one more aspect of personal care: sex. We're going to talk about stuff that deals with nasty, dirty, fun things and how to keep doing your dirty, nasty, fun things without harming any animals in the process. If talk of sex bothers you, stop being such a prude. Ah, we're just kidding. Seriously, if you have delicate sensibilities or you're a young'un, just flip to the next section.

Okay, with that said and out of the way, don't say we didn't warn you.

Condoms and Safe Sex Supplies

Earlier in the book, we complained that most latex condoms aren't vegan. Unfortunately, many latex condom producers use casein (a milk product) in their condoms. This is of course a gigantic pain in the ass, but the good news is that there are condoms out there that contain no animal products and are not tested on animals. Glyde, an Australian company, makes latex condoms, dams, and gloves that are truly vegan. The company claims that their condoms are produced using a patented "double dipping" method that makes them particularly strong without making them too thick. Nevertheless, the Glyde site (http://www.glydehealth.com) reminds you that "no condom can withstand sharp fingernails, diamond rings and metal body jewelry." You can even get Glyde condoms in three different sizes. The 53mm Glyde Ultra is for the "average" person, while the 49mm Slimfit and 56mm Maxis are for those at respective ends of the penis-size bell curve[7]. On top of all of this, Glyde condoms come in 5 "fun and fruity flavors" to make sex tasty as well as safe. Glyde also makes condoms for women, though we've never seen these for sale in the United States.

You can get Glyde condoms from many vegan stores, or you can order them from Veg Sex Shop (http://www.vegsexshop.com). The dams are available from the Veg Sex Shop or from http://www.sheerglydedams.com. Another brand, Condomi condoms (UK), are vegan but not readily available in the US; you can order online at http://www.condomi.com.

Lube

If you're using latex condoms and want some lube, you should always use a water-based lube since oil-based lubes can reduce the efficacy of latex condoms. Like many other manufactured health products, lubes can contain by-products of the animal slaughter industry (usually animal glycerin). Fortunately, there are plenty of vegan lubes on the market. You can find them at Toys in Babeland (http://babeland.com),

---

7. That's the most polite way we could figure out how to phrase that!

Veg Sex Shop, and other vegan stores. In addition to being animal free, many vegan lubes also contain more natural ingredients and/or are organic. There are so many brands that we wouldn't even know where to begin in recommending some. Look around and you'll find something good and slippery.

Leather

What is the vegan leather fetishist to do? Seriously, if you're into leather products but you abhor the cruelty involved in them, you can now find vegan substitutes for most of your leather and BDSM needs. Vegan Erotica (http://www.veganerotica.com) has tons of fake leather products that have the look, feel, and durability of the real thing. You can get spiked collars, belts, dildo harnesses and body harnesses, flogs, restraints, and just about anything else you'd need from there. On their website, Vegan Erotica says their products are made from Lorica, a synthetic leather that is permeable to water vapor, water repellent, machine-washable, and resistant to tearing, splitting, and scratching. In addition to these options, Veg Sex Shop also sells neoprene and rubber items that could be used for BDSM play (mostly cuffs and whips, at this writing).

Toys

Many sex toys are vegan, but "jelly rubber" items may contain mystery ingredients, so you cannot be sure that they're animal-free unless the manufacturer explicitly says they are. Most silicone toys are vegan, and silicone is the best material for sex toys anyway. The downside is that silicone toys aren't cheap, but they're worth the money because they're durable, easy to clean, and don't hold odors. Veg Sex Shop sells toys that are sure to be vegan, but you can also find all manner of silicone toys at Toys in Babeland. The nice part about both of these sites is that they're generally sex-positive and they're discreet.

Whatever you're into, odds are good you can find a vegan or animal-friendly way of expressing your desires; you may just have to use the Internet to get what you need (yet again).

Tattooing

There's simply no easy way to segue from sex toys into tattoos, so we're not even going to try. We thought before we closed out this chapter we'd briefly touch on tattooing and its implications for veganism. We both have tattoos, though Bob is something of a tattoo aficionado, and is planning on getting more tattoo work done in the future. If you haven't had a tattoo, yeah, they hurt (but not so bad). For some reason, tattooing is addictive. You might begin by thinking that you're only going to get one, and then a few years later, you could end up with your arms or back covered. It really surprises you, but if you have one tattoo, you'll probably want another.

The problem for vegans and tattoos comes in the ink. Most inks use glycerin as a carrier, and this glycerin is most often animal-based. Still, there are ways around this. If you know a good tattoo artist, odds are that you can ask her to get vegan ink for you in advance of an appointment, which will probably cost you extra. You may also be able to find vegan tattoo shops, but these are few and far between. In the end, it is up to you to decide how big a deal vegan tattoo ink is.

Because animal exploitation goes beyond animals being killed for food, ethical veganism also goes further than simply eliminating animal products from one's diet. Like other aspects of veganism, it can sometimes be challenging to make compassionate choices in a world that is structured around so much oppression. At times, it can be frustrating. You may feel that by eschewing leather, wool, down, and silk—on top of everything else—that you're the only person who cares about the plight of animals. This couldn't be further from the truth. If nothing else, this chapter shows that there are dedicated people who are promoting the abolition of animal slavery and exploitation through the development of vegan products, even in areas as diverse as sex toys and cosmetics. It might require a little extra planning and forethought, but before long, like other aspects of veganism, it becomes second nature. Best of all, it is completely worth it.

Books and Other Sources Mentioned in this Chapter

- Fact Sheet on Wool: *http://www.peta.org/mc/factsheet_display.asp?ID=55*

- *Empty Cages: Facing the Challenge of Animal Rights.* Regan, T. Rowman & Littlefield Publishers, Inc. (2004).

- *Mad Cowboy: Plain Truth from the Cattle Rancher Who Won't Eat Meat.* Lyman, H. F., & Merzer, G. Scribner. (2001).

- *Animal Ingredients A to Z : Third Edition.* E.G. Smith Collective. AK Press. (2004).

- *PeTA 2005 Shopping Guide For Caring Consumers: A Guide To Products That Are Not Tested On Animals (Shopping Guide for Caring Consumers).* People for the Ethical Treatment of Animals. Book Publishing Company (TN). (2004).

chapter six:

go vegan, stay vegan

People think vegans are freaks. If you don't have enough experience from your own day-to-day life to understand this, just have a quick look at anything in the popular media. Open *Newsweek,* or *The Guardian,* or even *The Village Voice.* Or just turn on Fox TV. If you actually look carefully enough in any of those venues, you'll find editorials, articles, or shows that paint vegetarians and vegans as freaks, either directly (*The Guardian* recently ran an opinion piece titled "Why I hate Vegetarians") or indirectly (as was the case with *Newsweek* and their coverage of the foie gras issue).

Maybe you're like us and unlucky enough to have suffered through two hours of the vegan episode of Fox TV's *Trading Spouses.* For those of you who avoid television—or who just avoid bad television—let us fill you in on the premise. Two families trade a spouse for a week, and hilarity ensues. Well, sometimes hilarity ensues. Fox doesn't pick two similar couples to trade spouses. After all, what fun would it be if, say, two blue-blood WASP families swapped spouses? They'd probably both end up at country clubs regardless, and the height of the social drama would probably be that one of the country clubs made their gin and tonics with Tanqueray instead of Bombay. Horrors.

To make the contrast completely evident even for slow TV viewers, Fox picks two families that live in completely different circumstances, often both materially and culturally. And so it was that Fox swapped mothers and wives from two different families on the show we watched. One family lived in the Louisiana swamp, had an alligator farm, and gave tours of the swamp for a living. The California family were vegans, as were most of their friends. The Louisiana swamp mom went to live in the California vegan house, and the California vegan went to live with the folks from the Bayou. Hilarity did indeed ensue.

The hilarity that ensued, however, made vegans look like pompous, judgmental assholes, and it frustrated us to no end. This might be because the vegan woman herself was pompous and judgmental, but that's probably why she was chosen for the show. The setup was such that the vegan would look like an ass while the Cajun mama appeared to be accepting, flexible, and giving. In one scene, she's getting ready to prepare a gumbo complete with alligator meat, sausages, and other creatures of the swamp when she sees a sign in the kitchen of her "new" home that states "No animals are to be consumed in this kitchen." Feeling that preparing her traditional Cajun gumbo would be an affront to the original "woman of the house," the Cajun mama of course decides to make a vegan gumbo. When she does, the vegan friends of the California family come over, act unappreciative of the vegan gumbo, and lecture the poor woman on animal rights.

On the flip side of the equation, the vegan mother in Louisiana lectures the family constantly on all manner of things. The kid doesn't brush his teeth well enough; they don't eat good food; they shouldn't be so mean to animals; they shouldn't drink so much soda; they need to give the kid more discipline. The vegan mother mindlessly lectures the Cajuns on how much land she saves by being a vegan, she talks about animal rights over food, and she tries to feed them vegan food, but with a hectoring tone about how much better it is for them. The vegan appears to be inflexible, and on top of it all, she is made to look like the contradictory fool that she is: in one scene, she actually hits a dog and rubs its face in urine for having peed on the floor. On top of all of this, she eats some fried alligator meat, and makes a huge deal out of it, but she ultimately justifies her decision by deciding that alligators aren't nice animals like cows. Seriously.

So we have a reality TV setup in which the Cajun meat eater is made to look flexible, accepting, and giving and the vegan is made to look judgmental, idiotic, and contradictory. This isn't an accident. The vegan was surely chosen because of her high V-quotient. Couple her self-righteousness about veganism and animal rights with her overall judgmental and nasty self and you end up with someone who does a lot of work towards painting vegans as idiotic, contradictory, and self-righteous freaks. Sadly, we do know vegans like this, but they're a minority.

There's little doubt in our minds that Fox chose this vegan because she would help to play out a familiar script about how vegans behave. The vegan herself did a ton of objectionable things that made us cringe for all of vegan freakdom. She proselytized. She lectured. She bothered people. She acted self-righteous. She forced herself and her views on others in the most garish of ways. So don't get us wrong: we think the vegan on the show was despicable. But the downside of this is that it allowed a familiar stereotype of vegans and vegetarians more generally to be played out for all of America. For those couch potatoes who've never met a vegan, vegan now means "judgmental asshole" and nothing else. And sadly, many people live their lives using TV as an educator.

Fox's representation of vegans is like any popular media representation of any group, really. Don't you know that all Latinos are either janitors, maids, gardeners, or gangsters? Or that all blacks are poor? Or that all white people live in the suburbs? Or that all vegans are judgmental radical assholes?

Take a look around the popular media. It is okay to pick on vegetarians and animal rights advocates. People enjoy doing it, and being a mostly non-violent lot, we put up with it. We're the fodder for stand-up comedians, sitcoms, and reality TV lampooning. And if we're not being lampooned as fools, we're being painted as sissies, radicals, and/or terrorists. Male vegetarians are inevitably painted as "feminine" because we deny the very blood of other animals that is meant to invigorate us, make us dominant, and give us the bloodthirsty drive that the modern world supposedly demands of us as we sit on our asses in our cubicles. In a recent article on foie gras, *Newsweek* falls into this trap[1]. First, *Newsweek* uses tradition to justify the cruelty of foie gras. But then they dig into animal rights folks as kill-joy "food police" who want to deprive everyone else of this charming, historical delicacy built on torture. But the real kicker comes at the end of the article:

> "It's all a huge misunderstanding, in the view of Michael Ginor, an owner of Hudson Valley Foie Gras, the upstate New York farm that produces most of the estimated 420 tons (or 1.8 billion calories) of foie gras consumed in the United States annually. Force-feeding ducks with a tube "does sound atrocious," he admits, but he maintains that waterfowl, lacking the mammalian gag reflex, do not suffer from the process. "Foie gras is easy to attack: it's for the rich, it's unnecessary, it's vain. It can be seen as all those things. But it's been around for 5,000 years." And Charlie Trotter himself would be the last to deny how good it is. Its texture meltingly soft as a chocolate truffle, its flavor a mouth-filling meatiness and sweetness that helps justify humanity's million-year struggle to the top of the food chain. *Unless, of course, madame would prefer the vegetable reduction on her asparagus instead?*" [italics in original]

Here, the magazine reduces animal cruelty to a "huge misunderstanding," making animal rights activists look like sub-intellectual fools. And of course, the authors couldn't resist mentioning our "struggle to the top of the food chain" (another ridiculously inaccurate anti-vegan/ AR quip that we hear pretty often). Were we to chuck these authors into a cage with some hungry lions, we might not hear much about struggles to the top of any food chain. But we digress.

In the closing paragraph above, the authors get in two final blows: the first blow is that suffering is tasty, reinforcing the idea that our tastes trump all, regardless of what horrid measures must be taken to produce

---

1. "A Flap Over Foie Gras," May 2, 2005

those tastes. The second blow is the italicized bit about preferring "vegetable reduction." Note that the question is addressed to "madame." There's a subtle double-insult here in which women are presumed to be hysterical, sensitive, and soft (e.g., prone to "misunderstanding" as described above) and in which those who do care about animal rights are feminized. Of course, "sirs" would never want a vegetable reduction because "real men" love to kill shit and eat it. We want steak with our cigars, damn you! *Newsweek's* thinly veiled hack-job on vegetarians and animal rights advocates makes us look like feminized fools while promoting the thousands of years of suffering inherent in foie gras.

While on the one hand we're weak and starry-eyed fools who don't know any better, on the other, we're the terrorists in your own backyard who'd happily save animals while we'd kill researchers, brainwash your children, and burn down the local research lab. Radical tactics do have their place in any movement that aims for total liberation, but critics like to distort the aims of groups like the Animal Liberation Front (ALF)[2] and even mainstream groups like the HSUS and PeTA. In particular, it is worth noting that the ALF has pledged not to do violence to animals, both human and non-human, though they do not have a problem with property destruction. Whether this is acceptable or not is up to you; the point here is that regardless of your stance on the ALF and more radical tactics, *all* vegans are being painted as radical terrorists by groups that are actually involved in the exploitation of animals.

The point of this brief exercise in media analysis is to show you that you're always already set up to be the freak if you're vegan. It doesn't matter if you're the kindest, most polite, and least intrusive person in the world (though what fun would that be?). The conventional mass media already have you pegged as either a wuss, a terrorist, or a judgmental idiot. And in any case, the rest of the world sees you as a weirdo anyway, if only because you don't do things just like they do. We

---

2. If you're interested in the ALF, you need to run out—now—and buy a copy of *Terrorists or Freedom Fighters? Reflections on the Liberation of Animals*, edited by Steven Best and Anthony J. Nocella II. The foreword by Ward Churchill also kicks ass and takes names.

Americans pride ourselves on our proud, individual spirit, but that's all bullshit at the end of the day. What we really value are people who toe the line, don't ask too many questions, buy a lot of stuff (preferably on credit), and don't create too many problems. Vegans don't much toe the line, at least when it comes to what's accepted for animal exploitation. We also ask a lot of questions. You can't be a vegan unless you ask hard questions about where your food comes from. And of course, we create lots of problems. So try as hard as you might, you'll never be seen as "normal" by those around you, and if you're worried about that, we'd like to encourage you to rethink the value of actually *being normal.*

Love your inner vegan freak. Embrace it and nourish it. Don't hide what you are or change for anyone else. You have to live your ethics, and you can't live your life for others if you're going to be true to what you know is right.

~~~~~~

In the beginning of the book, we called the consciousness that comes along with veganism a "complex gift." If you are almost vegan or are already vegan, you've likely gotten there because you've come to understand the ethical dilemma of using animals for human ends. You may have suspected this all along, knowing something wasn't right, or maybe you only recently came to this kind of realization. It doesn't really matter. What does matter is that you understand that this consciousness is a powerful thing, and something you should nurture. Despite probably growing up in a culture where animals are treated as things, you've come to see things otherwise and understand the alternatives to animal exploitation, oppression, and slavery. This consciousness is too powerful to ignore, and the implications of knowing are too strong to walk away from. The problem, of course, comes when you have to deal with the other 99% of the world that refuses to see the truth of animal exploitation, and this is why we say that the consciousness that accompanies veganism is complex. It enables you to see what others won't, but in seeing differently than others, you're also seen differently.

Being seen differently means that life as a vegan will always have its share of annoyances, large and small; we'd be lying if we told you otherwise. At times, it is frustrating to live in a world systematically set up to disregard the lives of other beings, particularly when you see those beings as something other than yours to exploit. Despite the frustrations that inevitably come along with veganism, being an ethical vegan is completely worth the effort. We wrote this book because we wanted to help you deal with living in this world. We want you to be a happy, healthy, and freaky vegan. And on top of it all, *we want you to stay vegan.*

All of the time and energy we put into this book will be worth it to us if we can help even just a few of you become vegan or live as happier vegans. For us, it isn't about the money, or getting our names out there, or any of the reasons people normally write and promote books. Our goal is to get as many people as possible to be vegans, because we see this as one of the best initial steps to building a more compassionate world free of animal exploitation. Yes, it will be a long haul, but fighting for what is right is never easy.

People might call you crazy or freaky or weird for your ethical veganism and stance on animal rights. That's okay. Just remember this: they once thought that people who thought the earth was round were crazy too.

GO VEGAN.

STAY VEGAN.

xoxo,

BOB AND JENNA

appendix a:
25 things you can do to get involved

Other than becoming vegan, many people are at a loss of how they can become more involved in reducing animal suffering, because they might think it takes more time, money, or intestinal fortitude than they think they have. Activism, however, can take many forms, and even what we might consider to be small things can have a huge impact. Here's a list of a variety of ways that you can make a difference as a vegan. Think about your strengths and what you like to do, and put these to work in positive ways. (For us, it took the shape of writing this book!)

1. Adopt a dog or a cat from a shelter. Encourage others to do the same and to spay/neuter.

2. Volunteer at an animal shelter.

3. "Adopt" a farm animal from a farm sanctuary.

4. Donate your time or money to a farm sanctuary. Take your kids or friends to visit.

5. Support Compassion Over Killing (http://www.cok.net), Vegan Outreach (http://www.veganoutreach.org), or a similar organization. Visit their websites for great info.

6. Organize or volunteer at a Meatout event (http://www.meatout.org).

7. Have a vegan potluck.

8. Cook a vegan meal for your family or friends.

9. Organize a vegan group at your school or university (see our hints in Chapter 3).

10. Screen *The Witness, Peaceable Kingdom*, or another vegan-friendly movie. Have plenty of literature and vegan food available.

11. Write to your senators and congresspeople to support or challenge critical legislation, like the foie gras force-feeding bans.

12. Write a letter to the editor of your local newspaper about vegan or AR issues.

13. Write a letter to a company you know uses animal products or tests on animals, and urge them to stop. Suggest alternatives, like vegetable-based glycerin instead of animal-based.

14. Leaflet or table. Groups such as COK and Vegan Action have excellent guides as to how to go about leafletting and tabling efficiently, and they also offer pamphlets and brochures. (http://www.cok.net/lit/leafleting/php) (http://www.veganoutreach.org/advocacy/index.html)

15. Wear a shirt that proudly proclaims your veganism.

16. Hang informational flyers on your office door or cubicle walls, the door to your room, etc.

17. Put a vegan-inspired quote or a web address to your favorite pro-vegan web page in the signature file of your email. (Thanks to Vegan Outreach for suggestions 15-17).

18. Make your own t-shirts, buttons, stickers, or handmade vegan items and give/sell them to people.

19. Write a zine, comic, blog, etc. about being vegan or do a vegan cookzine.

20. Encourage a local restaurant to provide vegan options regularly on their menu. Thank them profusely if they come through. Similarly, when omnivorous family and friends go out of their way to make you vegan food or otherwise respect your cruelty-free preferences, let them know how much you appreciate it!

21. Read vegan-themed books (see Appendix B for suggestions) that interest you and pass these books on to others.

22. Subscribe to or find a copy of *Herbivore, VegNews,* and/or *Satya* to find out about vegan food, culture, events, and more ways to get involved.

23. Go to a vegetarian food fair, conference, or workshop.

24. Join a CSA (community supported agriculture), or frequent and support local farmer's markets. Look for organic farms in your area and buy locally when possible.

25. Put up a display or give a presentation at your local public library. (http://www.cok.net/lit/library.php)

appendix b:

resources

This list of resources is by no means exhaustive, but it will definitely start you off on the right foot. Some of these have already been mentioned in the rest of the book, but we list even more here. As you browse through the links and find information on the books we mention, we suggest you keep a list of your own bookmarks so you can easily go back to the sites you like. Also check our website at http://www.vegan-freak.com for new and updated links. If we overlooked your site or business, it wasn't anything personal; we only know so much of the web. If you want to be listed here in the next edition of our book, send us an email at resources@veganfreak.com. Though we can't promise to list everyone who writes, we will list most sites or resources that are explicitly of vegan interest. Sound fair?

Internet Resources

AR and Vegan Groups and Information

* Compassion Over Killing: *http://www.cok.net*

* Vegan Outreach: *http://www.veganoutreach.org*

* The Vegan Society (UK): *http://www.vegansociety.com/html/*

* The Vegetarian Resource Group: *http://www.vrg.org/*

* Vegetarians In Paradise (LA Veg Newsletter): *http://www.vegparadise.com/*
* Vegan Vanguard: *http://www.veganvanguard.com/*
* International Vegetarian Union: *http://www.ivu.org*
* In Defense of Animals: *http://idausa.org/*
* People for the Ethical Treatment of Animals (PeTA): *http://www.peta.org*

Farm Sanctuaries

* The Farm Sanctuary: *http://www.farmsanctuary.org*
* Poplar Springs Animal Sanctuary: *http://www.animalsanctuary.org/*
* OohMahNee Farm: *http://www.oohmahneefarm.org/index.shtml*
* Animal Acres: *http://www.animalacres.org/*
* Eastern Shore Chicken Sanctuary & Education Center: *http://www.bravebirds.org/*
* Lighthouse Farm Sanctuary: *http://www.lighthousefarmsanctuary.org/*

Vegan Health and Nutrition

* Physicians Committee for Responsible Medicine (PCRM): *http://www.pcrm.org*
* Dr. Neal Barnard (PCRM): *http://www.nealbarnard.org/*
* Veg For Life (Farm Sanctuary): *http://www.vegforlife.org/*
* Dr. Michael Greger: *http://www.drgreger.org/*
* McDougall Wellness Center: *http://www.drmcdougall.com/*
* Vegan Health: *http://www.veganhealth.org/*

Vegan Blogs and Forums

This list will change frequently as new blogs and forums come and go. Check our website for updates at www.veganfreak.com.

Blogs That Focus on Veganism and Animal Rights

* Vegan Freaks: *http://www.veganfreaks.org*

* Veg Blog: *http://www.vegblog.org/*

* The Smoking Vegan: *http://thesmokingvegan.blogspot.com/*

* Animal Writings: *http://www.animalwritings.com/*

* Vegan Chai: *http://quarterlifecrisis.typepad.com/*

* Vegan Momma: *http://www.veganmomma.com/blog*

* Erik's Diner (also podcast): *http://www.vegan.com/*

Blogs of Annotated News Stories

* Vegan Porn: *http://www.veganporn.com*

* An Animal-Friendly Life: *http://ananimalfriendlylife.com/*

* Meat Facts: *http://soyjoy.blogspot.com/*

Forums

* The Post Punk Kitchen Forum:
  http://www.postpunkkitchen.com/forum/index.php

* Vegan Represent: *http://www.veganrepresent.com/*

* The Vegan Forum: *http://veganforum.com/forums/index.php*

* Veggie Boards: *http://www.veggieboards.com/boards/*

* Wiki Veg (ok, not a forum per se, but a wiki):
  http://www.wikiveg.org/Welcome

Online Vegan Recipes and Cooking Information

* The Post Punk Kitchen: *http://www.theppk.com*

* VegWeb: *http://www.vegweb.com*

* Vegan Eat: *http://www.veganeat.org/*

* Random Girl Recipes: *http://www.randomgirl.com/recipes.html*
* Veg Cooking: *http://www.vegcooking.com/*
* The Vegan Chef: *http://www.veganchef.com/*
* Vegan Cooking: *http://www.vegancooking.com/*
* Vegan Mania: *http://www.veganmania.com/*

Veg•n Restaurant Guides

* Happy Cow: *http://www.happycow.net/*
* Veg Guide: *http://www.vegguide.org/*
* Vegetarian Resource Group:
  http://www.vrg.org/restaurant/index.htm
* Veg Dining: *http://www.vegdining.com/Home.cfm*
* Veg Eats: *http://www.vegeats.com/*

Information on Vegan Alcohol

* PeTA: *http://www.peta.org*
* Vegan Porn: *http://www.veganporn.com/booze.pl*
* Vegan beer list:
  http://www.btinternet.com/~p.g.h/vegan_beer_list.htm
* Vegan Vanguard: *http://www.veganvanguard.com/vegism/beer.html*
* Vegans are from Mars - vegan wine list:
  http://vegans.frommars.org/wine
* Vegetarian Network Victoria:
  http://www.vnv.org.au/AlcoholByName.htm

Vegan Miscellaneous

* Sarah Kramer (Cookbook author): *http://www.govegan.net*
* Tattoo & Body Modification Info:
  http://encyc.bmezine.com/?Vegan

Where to Buy Vegan Items Online

We've kept this list to sites where you can actually order online, rather than just find out info about a certain brand.

General vegan stores

These stores carry a range of vegan items, from food to shoes, buttons, t-shirts, vitamins, toiletries and beauty products, etc.

* Vegan Essentials: *http://www.veganessentials.com*

* Food Fight! Vegan Grocery: *http://www.foodfightgrocery.com*

* Pangea Vegan Products: *http://www.veganstore.com*

* Vegan Unlimited: *http://veganunlimited.com*

* The Vegetarian Site: *http://www.thevegetariansite.com/*

* A Different Daisy: *http://differentdaisy.com/*

* Cosmo's Vegan Shoppe: *http://www.cosmosveganshoppe.com/*

Vegan Clothing, Shoes, and Accessories

* Otsu Vegan Style: *http://www.veganmart.com*

* Alternative Outfitters: *http://www.alternativeoutfitters.com*

* Moo Shoes: *http://www.mooshoes.com*

* QueenBee Creations: *http://www.buyolympia.com/queenbee/*

* American Apparel: *http://americanapparel.net/*

* Freerangers (UK): *http://www.freerangers.co.uk/index2.htm*

* Vegetarian Shoes (UK): *http://www.vegetarian-shoes.co.uk/*

* Vegetarian Belts: *http://vegetarianbelts.com/*

* Drop Soul Organics: *http://www.dropsoul.com/*

* Via Vegan: *http://www.viavegan.com/*

* Vegan Wares (Australia): *http://www.veganwares.com/*

* M. Avery Designs: *http://maverydesigns.com/home.shtml*

* Herbivore Clothing: *http://herbivoreclothing.com/*

Not All Vegan, but Has a Vegan Selection

* Earth Shoes: *http://www.earth.us/index.asp*
* Zappos: *http://www.zappos.com*

Vegan Cosmetics, Toiletries, and Beauty Products

* Kiss My Face: *http://www.kissmyface.com/Index.pasp*
* Dirty Kitty Soap Works: *http://www.cleanvegan.com/index.htm*
* Crazy Rumors Lip Balm: *http://www.crazyrumors.com/*
* Planda Company: *http://www.plandacompany.com/*
* Estrella Soaps: *http://www.estrellasoap.com/*
* Ecco Bella: *http://www.eccobella.com*
* Aveda: *http://www.aveda.com*

Vegan Food

Don't forget that the general vegan stores above sell vegan foods too.

Baked Goods and Sweets

* Sticky Fingers Bakery: *http://stickyfingersbakery.com/*
* Allison's Gourmet: *http://allisonsgourmet.com/*
* Sun Flour Baking Company: *http://sunflourbaking.com*
* Simple Treats: *http://www.simpletreats.com/*
* Alternative Baking Company: *http://www.alternativebaking.com*
* Good Baker: *http://www.goodbaker.com/*
* Lagusta's Luscious Truffles: *http://www.lagustasluscious.com*
* Liz Lovely Cookies: *http://www.lizlovely.com/*
* Vermont Maple Syrup:
  http://www.vermontmaple.org/maple-by-mail.html

Dairy, Egg, and Meat replacements

* Follow Your Heart (Vegenaise®, Vegan Gourmet Cheese™): *http://www.followyourheart.com/*

* No Meat.Com (vegetarian, not all vegan): *http://www.nomeat.com/*

* May Wah (Asian-style fake meat galore): *http://www.vegieworld.com/*

* Lumen Foods (excellent veggie jerkey): *http://www.soybean.com/*

Vegan Dog and Cat Food

* Vegan Cats has a wide range of cat and dog food, plus starter kits and information on making your pets vegan: *http://www.vegancats.com/index.html*

* Evolution Diet: *http://www.petfoodshop.com/*

Vegan Sex Accessories

* Glyde Condoms: *http://www.glydehealth.com/*

* Condomi Condoms: *http://www.condomi.com*

* Toys in Babeland: *http://www.babeland.com*

* Vegan Erotica: *http://www.veganerotica.com*

* Veg Sex Shop: *http://www.vegsexshop.com*

DVDs

* Peaceable Kingdom: *http://www.tribeofheart.com*

* The Witness: *http://www.tribeofheart.com*

* Meat Your Meat: *http://www.meetyourmeat.com/*

* Super Size Me: *http://www.supersizeme.com*

Vegan-Related Magazines

* Herbivore: *http://herbivoreclothing.com/magazine.page.html*
* Veg News: *http://www.vegnews.com/*
* Satya: *http://www.satyamag.com/index.html*

Books

Even though we've put the titles of the books first for easy browsing, the books are listed alphabetically by author.

Animal Rights and Related Vegan Issues and Theory

* *The Pornography of Meat.* Adams, C. J. Continuum International Publishing Group. (2003).

* *The Sexual Politics of Meat: A Feminist-Vegetarian Critical Theory.* Adams, C. J., & Adams, C. Continuum International Publishing Group. (1999).

* *Hitler: Neither Vegetarian Nor Animal Lover.* Berry, R., & Rowe, M. Pythagorean Books. (2004).

* *Terrorists or Freedom Fighters?: Reflections on the Liberation of Animals.* Best, S., & Nocella, A. J., II. Lantern Books. (2004).

* *Slaughterhouse: The Shocking Story of Greed, Neglect, and Inhumane Treatment Inside the U.S. Meat Industry.* Eisnitz, G. A. Prometheus Books. (1997).

* *Rain Without Thunder: The Ideology of the Animal Rights Movement.* Francione, G. L. Temple University Press. (1996).

* *Animals, Property, and the Law (Ethics and Action).* Francione, G. L. Temple University Press. (1995).

* *Introduction to Animal Rights: Your Child or the Dog?* Francione, G. L., & Watson, A. Temple University Press. (2000).

* *Obligate Carnivore: Cats, Dogs, and What it Really Means to be Vegan.* Gillen, J. Steinhoist Books. (2003).

* *Mad Cowboy: Plain Truth from the Cattle Rancher Who Won't Eat Meat.*

Lyman, H. F., & Merzer, G. Scribner. (2001).

* *Meat Market: Animals, Ethics, And Money.* Marcus, E. Brio Press. (2005).

* *Vegan: The New Ethics of Eating, Revised Edition.* Marcus, E. Mc-Books Press. (2000).

* *An Unnatural Order: Why We Are Destroying The Planet and Each Other.* Mason, J. Lantern Books. (2005).

* *Eternal Treblinka: Our Treatment of Animals and the Holocaust.* Patterson, C. Lantern Books. (2002).

* *Empty Cages: Facing the Challenge of Animal Rights.* Regan, T. Rowman & Littlefield Publishers, Inc. (2004).

* *Defending Animal Rights.* Regan, T. University of Illinois Press. (2001).

* *The Case for Animal Rights.* Regan, T. University of California Press. (1985).

* *Beyond Beef : The Rise and Fall of the Cattle Culture.* Rifkin, J. Plume. (1993).

* *Diet for a New America: How Your Food Choices Affect Your Health, Happiness and the Future of Life on Earth.* Robbins, J. H.J. Kramer. (1998).

* *Fast Food Nation: The Dark Side of the All-American Meal.* Schlosser, E. Perennial. (2002).

* *Animal Liberation.* Singer, P. Ecco. (2001).

* *The Dreaded Comparison: Human and Animal Slavery.* Spiegel, M. Mirror Books. (1997).

* *Animal Others: On Ethics, Ontology, and Animal Life (SUNY Series in Contemporary Continental Philosophy).* Steeves, H. P., & Regan, T. State University of New York Press. (1999).

Vegan Health, Nutrition, and Diet

* *Food for Life: How the New Four Food Groups Can Save Your Life.* Barnard, N. Three Rivers Press (CA). (1994).

* *Eat Right, Live Longer : Using the Natural Power of Foods to Age Proof Your Body.* Barnard, N. Harmony. (1995).

* *The China Study : The Most Comprehensive Study of Nutrition Ever Conducted and the Startling Implications for Diet, Weight Loss and Long-Term Health.* Campbell, T. C., & Campbell, T.M. II. Benbella Books. (2005).

* *Diet for a Dead Planet: How the Food Industry Is Killing Us.* Cook, C. D. New Press. (2004).

* *Becoming Vegan: The Complete Guide to Adopting a Healthy Plant-Based Diet.* Davis, B., & Melina, V. Book Publishing Company (TN). (2000).

* *Carbophobia: The Scary Truth About America's Low-carb Craze.* Greger, M., M.D. Lantern Books. (2005).

* *The McDougall Program for Women: What Every Woman Needs to Know to Be Healthy for Life.* McDougall, J. A., McDougall, M. A., Plume. (2000).

* *The Food Revolution: How Your Diet Can Help Save Your Life and Our World.* Robbins, J., & Ornish, M. D., Dean. Conari Press. (2001).

* *The Vegan Diet As Chronic Disease Prevention: Evidence Supporting the New Four Food Groups.* Saunders, K. Lantern Books. (2003).

* *Raising Vegetarian Children : A Guide to Good Health and Family Harmony.* Stepaniak, J., & Melina, V. McGraw-Hill. (2002).

* *World Peace Diet: Eating for Spiritual Health and Social Harmony.* Tuttle, W. Lantern Books. (2005).

Vegan Miscellaneous

* *Living Among Meat Eaters: The Vegetarian's Survival Handbook.* Adams, C. J. Continuum International Publishing Group. (2003).

* *The Inner Art of Vegetarianism : Spiritual Practices for Body.* Adams, C. J. Booklight. (2000).

* *Animal Ingredients A to Z : Third Edition.* E.G. Smith Collective. AK Press. (2004).

* *PeTA 2005 Shopping Guide For Caring Consumers: A Guide To Products That Are Not Tested On Animals (Shopping Guide for Caring Consumers).* People for the Ethical Treatment of Animals. Book Publishing Company (TN). (2004).

* *The Vegan Sourcebook.* Stepaniak, J. McGraw Hill. (2000).

Veg*n Dining Guides

* *The Vegan Guide To New York City.* Berry, R., & Suzuki, C. A. Ethical Living. (2004).

* *Veg Out Vegetarian Guide* Series. Guidebooks for New York City, San Francisco Bay Area, Southern California, Washington, D.C., Seattle and Portland, Chicago, Denver and Salt Lake City, and it looks like more are on the way.

* *Vegetarian Restaurants and Natural Food Stores in the U. S. : A Comprehensive Guide to Over 2500 Vegetarian Eateries.* Howley, J. Torchlight Publishing. (2002).

Cookbooks

We haven't tried all of these, but everyone has different tastes when it comes to cookbooks and cooking, so we listed a bunch. We put a † next to the ones we can personally recommend.

Good, general all-vegan cookbooks

* †*The Garden of Vegan : How It All Vegan Again!.* Barnard, T., & Kramer, S. Arsenal Pulp Press. (2003).

* *The Everyday Vegan.* Burton, D. Arsenal Pulp Press. (2001).

* *Vive le Vegan! : Simple, Delectable Recipes for the Everyday Vegan Family.* Burton, D. Arsenal Pulp Press. (2004).

* *125 Best Vegan Recipes.* Chuck, M. E., & Gurney, B. Robert Rose.

(2005).

* *The Accidental Vegan*. Gartenstein, D. Crossing Press. (2000).

* *The Complete Vegan Cookbook: Over 200 Tantalizing Recipes, Plus Plenty of Kitchen Wisdom for Beginners and Experienced Cooks*. Geiskopf-Hadler, S., & Toomay, M. Three Rivers Press. (2001).

* *Venturesome Vegetarian Cooking : Bold Flavors for Meat- and Dairy-Free Meals*. Hirsch, J. M., Hirsch, M., & Mackey, J. Surrey Books. (2004).

* *The Chicago Diner Cookbook*. Kaucher, J. A. Book Publishing Company (TN). (2002).

* *The Voluptuous Vegan : More Than 200 Sinfully Delicious Recipes for Meatless, Eggless, and Dairy-Free Meals*. Kornfeld, M., Minot, G., & Hamanaka, S. Clarkson Potter. (2000).

* *La Dolce Vegan!: Vegan Livin' Made Easy*. Kramer, S. Arsenal Pulp Press. (2005).

* †*How It All Vegan!: Irresistible Recipes for an Animal-Free Diet*. Kramer, S., & Barnard, T. Arsenal Pulp Press. (1999).

* *Vegan Cooking For One*. Leneman, L. Thorsons Publishers. (2000).

* †*Teany Book: Stories, Food, Romance, Cartoons and, of Course, Tea*. Moby, Tisdale, K. Studio. (2005).

* †*Vegan with a Vengeance : 125 Delicious, Cheap, Animal-Free, Logo-Free Recipes That Rock*. Moskowitz, I. C. Marlowe & Company. (2005).

* †*The Native Foods Restaurant Cookbook*. Petrovna, Tanya. Shambhala. (2003).

* *The Peaceful Palate: Fine Vegetarian Cuisine*. Raymond, J. Book Publishing Company (TN). (1996).

* †*Vegan Planet : 400 Irresistible Recipes with Fantastic Flavors from Home and Around the World*. Robertson, R. Harvard Common Press. (2003).

* *The Vegetarian Meat and Potatoes Cookbook*. Robertson, R. Harvard

Common Press. (2002).

* *The New Vegan Cookbook: Innovative Vegetarian Recipes Free of Dairy, Eggs, and Cholesterol.* Sass, L. J., & Weaver, J. Chronicle Books. (2001).

* *The New Now and Zen Epicure: Gourmet Vegan Recipes for the Enlightened Palate.* Schinner, M. N. Book Publishing Company (TN). (2001).

* *Vegan Vittles: Recipes Inspired by the Critters of Farm Sanctuary.* Stepaniak, J. Book Publishing Company (TN). (1996).

* *Meatless Meals for Working People: Quick and Easy Vegetarian Recipes.* Wasserman, D., & Stahler, C. Vegetarian Resource Group. (2001).

* *Vegan Cookbook: Over 90 Mouthwatering New Dairy Free Recipes for All Occasions.* Weston, T., & Bishop, Y. Hamlyn. (2004).

Good Cookbooks When You Want Something Fancy

* *Horizons: The Cookbook.* Landau, R., & Jacoby, K. Book Publishing Company (TN). (2005).

* *The Angelica Home Kitchen: Recipes and Rabble Rousings from an Organic Vegan Restaurant.* McEachern, L., & Taylor, J. B. Ten Speed Press. (2003).

* *†The Candle Cafe Cookbook : More Than 150 Enlightened Recipes from New York's Renowned Vegan Restaurant.* Pierson, J., Potenza, B., & Scott-Goodman, B. Clarkson Potter. (2003).

* *Vegan World Fusion Cuisine...The Cookbook and Wisdom Work from the Chefs of the Blossoming Lotus Restaurant With a Special Foreword by Dr. Jane Goodall, Second Edition.* Reinfeld, M., & Rinaldi, B. (2004).

* *The Artful Vegan: Fresh Flavors from the Millennium Restaurant.* Tucker, E., Enloe, B., Comet, R., & Pearce, A. Ten Speed Press. (2003).

* *Millennium Cookbook: Extraordinary Vegetarian Cuisine.* Tucker, E., Westerdahl, J., & Weiss, S. Ten Speed Press. (1998).

Regional and Specialized Cookbooks

* *Flavors of Korea: Delicious Vegetarian Cuisine (Healthy World Cuisine).*
  Coultrip-Davis, D., Davis, D., & Ramsay, Y. S. Book Publishing
  Company (TN). (1998).

* *Authentic Chinese Cuisine: For the Contemporary Kitchen.* Grogan, B. C.
  Book Publishing Company (TN). (2000).

* *Nonna's Italian Kitchen: Delicious Homestyle Vegan Cuisine (Healthy
  World Cuisine).* Grogan, B. C. Book Publishing Company (TN).
  (1998).

* †*The Mediterranean Vegan Kitchen: Meat-Free, Egg-Free, Dairy-Free
  Dishes from the Healthiest Place Under the Sun.* Klein, D. HP Books.
  (2001).

* *Japanese Cooking - Contemporary & Traditional.* Schinner, M. N., &
  Schinner, M. N. Book Publishing Company (TN). (1999).

* †*The Ultimate Uncheese Cookbook: Delicious Dairy-Free Cheeses and
  Classic "Uncheese" Dishes.* Stepaniak, J. Book Publishing Company
  (TN). (2003).

* †*Vegan Deli.* Stepaniak, J. Book Publishing Company (TN).
  (2001).

* †*The Nutritional Yeast Cookbook: Recipes Using Red Star Vegetarian
  Support Formula.* Stepaniak, J., & Publishing, B. Book Publishing
  Company (TN). (1997).

Desserts and Baking

* *Great Good Desserts Naturally!.* Costigan, F. Good Cakes Publica-
  tions. (2000).

* *More Great Good Desserts!: Secrets of Sensational Sin-free Vegan Sweets.*
  Costigan, F. Book Pub Co. (2005).

* *Sinfully Vegan: Over 140 Decadent Desserts to Satisfy Every Vegan's
  Sweet Tooth.* Dieterly, L. Marlowe & Company. (2003).

* *Sweet and Natural: More Than 120 Sugar-Free and Dairy-Free Desserts.*

McCarty, M. St. Martin's Press. (2001).

* *†Lickin' the beaters: low fat vegan desserts.* Moffat, S. Mr. Pither Cycling Tour Concoctions. (2003).

* *Vice Cream: Over 70 Sinfully Delicious Dairy-Free Delights.* Rogers, J. Ten Speed Press. (2004).

Mostly Vegetarian Cookbooks (but swith some good vegan or veganizable recipes)

* *†Lord Krishna's Cuisine: The Art of Indian Vegetarian Cooking.* Devi, Y. Dutton Books. (1987).

* *†3 Bowls : Vegetarian Recipes from an American Zen Buddhist Monastery.* Farrey, S. E., & O'Hara, N. Houghton Mifflin. (2000).

* *†Madhur Jaffrey's World Vegetarian : More Than 650 Meatless Recipes from Around the World.* Jaffrey, Madhur. Clarkson Potter. (2002).

* *†Madhur Jaffrey's World-of-the-East Vegetarian Cooking.* Jaffrey, Madhur. Knopf. (1981).

index

About the Authors

Bob Torres received his PhD and MS degrees from Cornell University in Development Sociology. Bob also has a BA in Philosophy and a BS in agricultural science from Penn State. He is currently a professor of sociology at a small liberal arts college in upstate New York, where he teaches classes on globalization, international development, and political economy. Occasionally, they even let him teach on animal rights issues.

Jenna Torres attended Cornell University for her PhD and MA degrees in Spanish Linguistics, and received a BA in Spanish and a BS in Plant Science from Penn State. Currently a visiting professor of modern languages at the same small liberal arts college, her specialty is in linguistics and second language acquisition, and she teaches classes on Spanish.

Bob and Jenna live in the northern foothills of the Adirondacks with their cat Michi and their crazy dog Mole (as in the Mexican sauce, pronounced "mole-lay").

Colophon

This text was typeset in Adobe Garamond. Dingbats at the top of each chapter are from the Tombats font sets, done by Tom Murphy (http://fonts.tom7.com). Chapter titles and headers are done in Formata Bold Condensed.

Music used during the production of this book: Sleater-Kinney, *The Woods*; Bloc Party, *Silent Alarm*; Sasha, *Involver*; Death Cab for Cutie, *John Byrd EP*; Satoshi Tomiie, *Global Underground NuBreed 006*; LCD Soundsystem, *LCD Soundsystem*; Arcade Fire; *Funeral*.

We'd never have finished this book without cashew butter sandwiches, Tofutti cuties, and walks in the local wooded areas with our dog Mole.

Have a freaky friend?
Order 'em a copy of

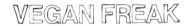

being vegan in a non-vegan world

Copy or rip out this page, fill it out, enclose payment,
send it off and we'll get your copy in the mail.

Name: _____

Shipping Address*: _____

_____

_____

*US shipping addresses only; visit our website for international orders.

Email: _____

___ Please add me to Tofu Hound Press/Vegan Freak email list

Enclose a money order or check made payable to "Tofu Hound Press" for $15.95
(US-shipping and handling included). New York State Residents, please enclose $16.86
(shipping, handling, and sales tax included).

Put this form and your payment in an envelope, and mail it to:

Tofu Hound Press

PO Box 276

Colton, NY 13625

For faster service order direct on the Internet:

www.tofuhound.com

Don't forget to visit
veganfreak.com
for updates to the resources in this book!

Printed in the United States
69888LV00002B/1087-1113